Workbook for

Lippincott's Essentials for Nursing Assistants

Second Edition

PAMELA J. CARTER, RN, BSN, MEd, CNOR
Program Coordinator/Instructor
School of Health Professions
Davis Applied Technology College
Kaysville, Utah

Wolters Kluwer | Lippincott Williams & Wilkins
Health
Philadelphia · Baltimore · New York · London
Buenos Aires · Hong Kong · Sydney · Tokyo

Acquisitions Editor: Elizabeth Nieginski
Development Editors: Melanie Cann, Season Evans
Director of Nursing Production: Helen Ewan
Senior Managing Editor/Production: Erika Kors
Design: Holly McLaughlin
Art Director, Illustration: Brett MacNaughton
Manufacturing Coordinator: Karin Duffield
Production Services/Compositor: Aptara, Inc.

2nd Edition

Copyright © 2010 Wolters Kluwer Health | Lippincott Williams & Wilkins.

9 8 7 6 5 4

Printed in the United States of America

Library of Congress Cataloging-in-Publication Data

Carter, Pamela J.
    Workbook for Lippincott's Essentials for Nursing Assistants / Pamela J. Carter.—2nd
ed.
        p. ; cm.
    ISBN 978-1-60547-003-0 (alk. paper)
    1. Nurses' aides   I. Carter, Pamela J. Lippincott's essentials for nursing assistants.
II. Title.
    RT84.C37 2007 Suppl.
    610.7306'98—dc22

                                                        2008032360

Preface

The *Workbook for Lippincott's Essentials for Nursing Assistants, 2nd edition,* developed alongside *Lippincott's Essentials for Nursing Assistants, 2nd edition,* with the aid of an instructional design team, is designed to help students internalize and apply the important concepts and facts presented in the textbook. Students will benefit from first reading the assignment in the textbook and then completing the corresponding workbook assignment. This approach allows students to review and reinforce the information that they have just read. In addition, after working on the workbook assignment, students who are having difficulty understanding the information presented in the textbook will know what type of questions they need to ask in class the following day. This ability to recognize areas of difficulty helps students to better utilize instruction time.

A UNIQUE ORGANIZATION

The organization of each chapter in the *Workbook for Lippincott's Essentials for Nursing Assistants, 2nd edition,* follows the same organization as the corresponding chapter in *Lippincott's Essentials for Nursing Assistants, 2nd edition.* This unique organization enhances flexibility with regard to assignments—it is easy to assign all, or just part of, a workbook chapter, according to the needs of your particular curriculum. In addition, this unique organization allows students to identify particular areas of difficulty where more clarification and review is needed. **Key Learning Points,** derived from the learning objectives in the textbook, are given for each sub-topic within the chapter and help the student to easily identify the concepts that are being reviewed and reinforced.

ACTIVITIES DESIGNED TO APPEAL TO DIFFERENT TYPES OF LEARNERS

This workbook uses several different types of activities to help students internalize and apply the information in the textbook. A wide variety of activities is important for appealing to students with different learning styles. Variety also helps to keep students engaged in the assignment. Some of the activity types that you will find in this workbook include:

- **Multiple-choice questions:** Select the single best answer from four choices.
- **Fill-in-the-blanks:** Complete a phrase or sentence.
- **Think About It!** Write a short response to a thought-provoking "what if?" scenario.
- **True or false?** Identify the true statements and correct the false ones.
- **Matching:** Match the terms or pictures to their descriptions.
- **Crossword puzzles:** Decipher the clues to complete the puzzle.
- **Word jumbles:** Use the clues to rearrange scrambled letters and reveal key vocabulary words.
- **Labeling:** Fill in the missing labels on a key piece of artwork.
- **Sequencing:** Put the steps of a procedure or process in the correct order.
- **Identification:** Recognize the phrases or sentences that apply to each situation.

Many workbooks rely heavily on multiple-choice questions. Although multiple-choice questions are important for helping students to prepare for the certification exam, the goal of this workbook is to help prepare students for what comes after the exam. We want students to develop a depth of understanding of this material that will serve them well in their clinical practice, long after the exam is over. Our goal is to help promote good problem-solving abilities and more of a "working" application of the material. Instructors wishing to provide their students with additional practice in answering multiple-choice questions can create worksheets and practice tests using the Test Generator questions provided on the *Instructor's Resource DVD for Lippincott's Essentials for Nursing Assistants*, 2nd edition and on thePoint, a web-based course and content management system (http://thepoint.lww.com/carteressentials2e).

OTHER KEY FEATURES

In addition to a variety of activities designed to reinforce the information in Chapters 1 through 30 and Appendix B ("Introduction to the Language of Health Care") of *Lippincott's Essentials for Nursing Assistants*, 2nd edition, this workbook contains:

■ **Procedure checklists.** These checklists are very useful during the laboratory portion of the course, when students are practicing the procedures they have just learned.

■ **Pam's pearls:** Scattered throughout the workbook, these words of advice and encouragement from the author serve to reinforce key concepts and remind students of the very important role they will play in providing patient and resident care.

Preventing the complications of immobility through frequent repositioning and transferring is a major responsibility of the nursing assistant!

Answers to the activities in the *Workbook for Lippincott's Essentials for Nursing Assistants*, 2nd edition, are provided on the *Instructor's Resource DVD for Lippincott's Essentials for Nursing Assistants*, 2nd edition. The answers may be given to the student at the instructor's discretion.

It is our sincere hope that students will find completing assignments from the *Workbook for Lippincott's Essentials for Nursing Assistants*, 2nd edition to be fun as well as educational. As always, we welcome and appreciate feedback from our readers.

Pamela J. Carter
Lippincott Williams & Wilkins

Acknowledgments

We wish to thank Season Evans, Joellen Shumway, and the instructional design teams at LearningMate Content Solutions for their assistance during the development of this workbook.

Contents

CHAPTER 1

The Health Care System

A HOLISTIC APPROACH TO HEALTH CARE

Key Learning Points

- The benefits of a holistic approach to health care the person receiving care
- How the health care team works together to provide holistic care
- The words *holistic* and *health care team*

Activity A *Fill in the blanks using the words given in parentheses.*

(family, physical, health, emotional)

1. A holistic approach to health care takes into consideration the person's _physical_ and _emotional_ needs.

2. In the past, the "_family_ doctor" could provide holistic care to his patients as he was familiar with each person as an individual.

3. Today, patients benefit from the knowledge and expertise of several people who are part of the _health_ care team that provides holistic care.

Activity B *Place an "X" next to the statements that are true about the health care team.*

1. _____ The doctor is more important than any other member of the health care team.

2. _X_ The health care team is made up of many people with different types of knowledge and skill levels.

3. _X_ The job of each member of the health care team is as important as that of any other member.

Activity C *Mark each statement as either "true" (T) or "false" (F). Correct the false statements.*

1. (T) F A health care team provides holistic care.

2. T (F) The person's emotional needs are not considered during treatment.

3. (T) F The family doctor was able to provide holistic care to his patients.

Activity D *Look at the figure and answer the question following it.*

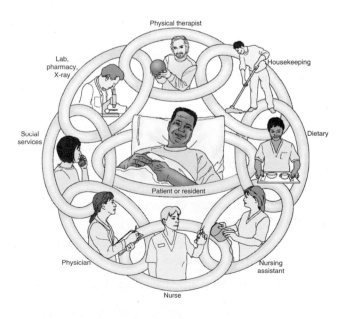

1

1. In a health care setting, who is always the focus of the health care team's efforts?

    a. The physician
    b. The housekeeping staff
    c. The patient or resident
    d. Social services

⬤ Health care is provided by a team of people, each with different areas of expertise and job responsibilities. As a nursing assistant, you are a critical member of the health care team!

HEALTH CARE ORGANIZATIONS

Key Learning Points

- Types of health care organizations
- Structure of health care organization

Activity A *Match the types of people you care for, given in Column A, with their descriptions, given in Column B.*

Column A

_C_ 1. A client

_a_ 2. A patient

_b_ 3. A resident

Column B

a. A person who is receiving health care in a hospital.

b. A person who is living in a long-term care facility.

c. A person who is receiving care in his or her own home.

⬤ As a nursing assistant you care for people who are sick, injured, or unable to care for themselves.

Activity B *Fill in the blanks using the words given in parentheses.*

(hospice, assisted-living facility, hospital, home health care, sub-acute care unit, long-term care facility)

1. This organization focuses on rehabilitation and helping the person to move from hospital care to home care. _Sub-acute care unit_

2. This organization provides inpatient or outpatient care for people with acute medical or surgical conditions. _Hospital care unit_

3. This organization provides care for people who are unable to care for themselves at home, but do not need to be hospitalized. _long term care facility_

4. This organization provides skilled care for people of all ages, with different medical needs, in the person's own home. _home health care_

5. This organization focuses on providing pain relief to the dying and providing emotional and spiritual support for both the dying person and the family. _Hospice_

6. This facility provides care for people who need limited help with medications, transportation, meals, and housekeeping. _assisted living facility_

Activity C *Most health care organizations are set up in a way similar to that shown in the chart below. Fill in the blank boxes and complete the chart.*

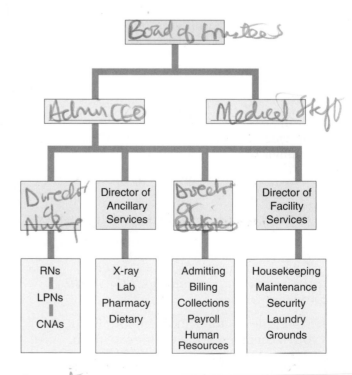

PATIENTS, RESIDENTS, AND CLIENTS

Key Learning Points

- The need for health care
- Classification of people according to their health care needs

Activity A *To make providing health care more efficient, the health care industry groups people according to their ages, illnesses, medical conditions, or special health care needs. Use the clues to complete the crossword puzzle.*

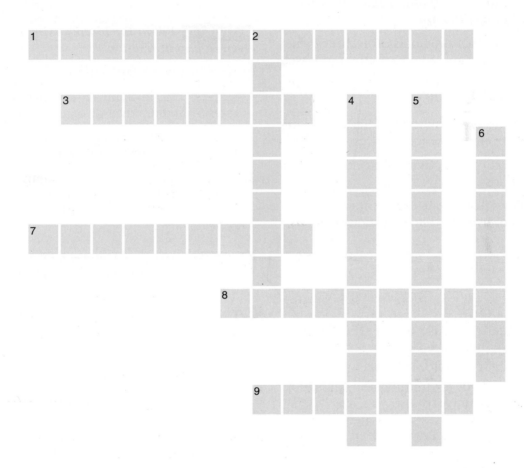

ACROSS

1. Patients who are receiving therapy to restore their highest level of functioning
3. Patients who do not need total care provided by a hospital, but are not quite ready to return home
7. Patients who are children and adolescents
8. People who are 75 years or older
9. Patients who have an illness or condition that is treated with methods other than surgery, such as medication, physical therapy, or radiation

DOWN

2. Type of care required by patients who are critically ill and require highly skilled monitoring and care
4. Patients with mental health disorders
5. Patients who are pregnant or have just given birth
6. Patients with conditions that are treated by surgery

GOVERNMENT REGULATION OF THE HEALTH CARE SYSTEM

Key Learning Points

- How government regulations affect the health care system
- The words *OBRA* and *OSHA*

Activity A *Place an "X" next to the statements that are true about the role of the government in health care.*

1. _____ Ensures that providers of health care are properly trained and able to do their jobs well

2. _____ Ensures that quality health care is available to select groups of people

3. _____ Ensures that providers of health care are protected from on-the-job injuries

4. _____ Monitors the activity of health care organizations

5. _____ Allows health care organizations to skip standards of hygiene that are tedious to follow

Activity B *Place an "X" next to each correct answer to the following questions.*

1. The Omnibus Budget Reconciliation Act (OBRA) of 1987 ensures:

   _____ a. Quality care for people who live in long-term care facilities

   _____ b. Quality care for nursing assistants

   _____ c. Standards for training and evaluation of nursing assistants

2. The Occupational Safety and Health Act of 1970:

   _____ a. Guarded the health of the government

   _____ b. Established safety and health standards for the workplace

   _____ c. Developed the Occupational Safety and Health Administration standards

PAYING FOR HEALTH CARE

Key Learning Points

- Paying for health care
- Purpose of the Minimum Data Set (MDS)
- The words *Medicare* and *Medicaid*

 Health care can be expensive. Insurance can help to reduce these costs for the individual.

Activity A *Fill in the blanks using the words given in parentheses.*

(private, managed care, group)

1. _____ insurance is purchased at group rates by an employer or corporation.

2. _____ insurance is purchased privately by individuals using their own funds.

3. _____ _____ systems help to deliver health care to people who need it by arranging contacts with various health care providers.

Activity B *Mark each statement as either "true" (T) or "false" (F). Correct the false statements.*

1. T F   Medicare is paid for by individuals.

2. T F   Younger people with disabilities may be eligible for Medicare.

3. T F   Only people who are 65 years or older with low income are eligible for Medicare.

4. T F   Medicaid is an insurance plan funded by the federal government.

5. T F   Medicaid helps people with low incomes to pay for health care.

6. T F   Elderly people and the disabled are eligible for Medicaid, especially if they have limited incomes.

7. T F   To receive Medicaid reimbursement, a facility need not always be approved by the state agency.

Activity C *Place an "X" next to the statements that are true about Medicare reimbursement.*

1. _____ Long-term health care facilities do not need to complete a Minimum Data Set report to receive Medicare reimbursements.

2. _____ Information such as the person's weight or bowel and bladder habits is recorded regularly as part of the MDS report.

3. _____ It is not necessary to record the care given to patients and residents.

4. _____ Proper recording of the care provided is necessary to ensure that the health care facility continues to receive Medicare reimbursements.

Activity D *Fill in the blanks using the words given in parentheses.*

(Minimum Data Set, Medicare, Medicaid)

1. _____ is a federally funded insurance plan for people who are 65 years and older and for some disabled people who are younger.

2. A _____ _____ _____ is a record of information such as the person's weight, bowel and bladder habits, and ability to care for ones self.

3. _____ is a federally funded insurance plan for people with low incomes.

CHAPTER 2

The Nursing Assistant's Job

EDUCATION OF THE NURSING ASSISTANT

Key Learning Points

- The Omnibus Budget Reconciliation Act (OBRA) requirements for nursing assistant training
- Certification process
- Contents of the registry
- The words *competency evaluation, reciprocity,* and *registry*

Activity A *Place an "X" next to the statements that are true about the OBRA requirement for nursing assistant training.*

1. _____ A minimum of 75 hours of training is required.

2. _____ Training consists of only classroom lectures.

3. _____ Training involves only hands-on practice of skills.

4. _____ Training involves supervised experience in an actual health care setting.

5. _____ Training includes classroom lectures and hands-on practice of skills.

Activity B *Place an "X" next to the information that does NOT appear in the registry.*

1. _____ Full name

2. _____ Home address

3. _____ Social Security number

4. _____ Date of birth

5. _____ Date the competency evaluation was passed

6. _____ Marital status

7. _____ Reported incidents of resident abuse or neglect, or theft of resident property

Activity C *Fill in the blanks using the words given in parentheses.*

(competency evaluation, three, reciprocity, registry)

1. An examination that must be passed at the end of the nursing assistant training course to obtain certification

   _____

2. The principle by which one state recognizes the validity of a license or certification granted by another state

   _____

3. An official record maintained by the state of the people who have successfully completed the nursing assistant training program

   _____

4. The number of chances OBRA specifies that you will have to complete the evaluation successfully

   _____

THE NURSING ASSISTANT AS A MEMBER OF THE NURSING TEAM

Key Learning Points

- The members of the nursing team, and the role of each team member
- How the nursing process is used to create the nursing care plan
- The delegation process as it relates to the nursing assistant
- The "five rights" of delegation
- The words *nursing plan of care, nursing process, delegate,* and *scope of practice*

Activity A *Fill in the blanks using the words given in parentheses.*

(head nurse, registered nurse, director of nursing, licensed practical nurse, charge nurse, licensed vocational nurse)

1. The nursing team consists of at least a nurse and a nursing assistant. A nurse

   can either be a _____ _____

   _____ (LPN), or a _____

   _____ (RN). In some states, an LPN

   is also referred to as a _____

   _____ _____ (LVN). A nursing

   team could also include a _____

   _____, whose duty involves supervising other nurses during a shift, and a

   _____ _____, who heads a department or section. An RN who directs all the nursing care within a health care

   organization is called a _____

   _____ (DON).

Activity B *Match the types of nursing care, given in Column A, with their descriptions, given in Column B.*

Column A

_C_ **1.** Primary nursing

_A_ **2.** Functional (modular) nursing

____ **3.** Team nursing

Column B

a. Each member of the nursing team carries out the same assigned task for all patients or residents.

b. An RN determines all of the nursing needs for the patients or residents assigned to the team

and assigns tasks according to each team member's skills and level of responsibility.

c. One nurse is assigned several patients or residents and is responsible for planning and carrying out all aspects of care for those people.

Activity C *Fill in the blanks using the words given in parentheses. Also, write down the correct order of the steps in the boxes provided below.*

[planning, diagnosis, implementation, assessment, evaluation]

Mrs. Chang has been admitted to the long-term care facility where you work because her Alzheimer's disease has progressed to the point where she is no longer able to manage many basic activities, such as bathing, dressing, and using the toilet. Susan, the nursing team leader, is responsible for preparing a nursing care plan for Mrs. Chang. Susan will use the nursing process to prepare this plan. The nursing process is organized into a series of steps.

1. _____ The nursing team carries out the interventions detailed in the nursing care plan.

2. _____ The nursing team checks the effectiveness of the plan and revises it as necessary.

3. _____ The nurse describes the problems that Mrs. Chang is having, as well as the cause of the problems.

4. _____ The nurse examines Mrs. Chang and asks questions about her abilities, habits, and needs.

5. _____ The nurse makes a plan for Mrs. Chang's care.

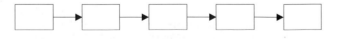

Activity D *Mark each statement as either "true" (T) or "false" (F). Correct the false statements.*

1. **T F** "Scope of practice" refers to the range of tasks that a nursing assistant is morally permitted to do.

2. T F By delegating a task, a nurse gives a nursing assistant permission to perform the task on his or her behalf.

3. T F Tasks such as assessment, planning, and evaluating can be delegated to nursing assistants.

4. T F A nursing assistant can take a person's vital signs and record this information on the person's chart.

5. T F A nursing assistant is qualified to interpret the data on the person's chart.

Activity E *The National Council of State Boards of Nursing (NCSBN) has developed guidelines, called the "five rights" of delegation, to help nurses effectively delegate tasks. Match the "rights," given in Column A, with their guidelines, given in Column B.*

Column A

_____ **1.** The right task

_____ **2.** The right circumstance

_____ **3.** The right person

_____ **4.** The right direction

_____ **5.** The right supervision

Column B

a. Will the nurse be available to supervise or answer questions?

b. Will the nurse be able to give the nursing assistant clear directions regarding how to perform the task?

c. What are the needs of the patient or resident at this time?

d. Can this task be delegated?

e. Does the nursing assistant have the right training and experience to safely complete the task?

Activity F *Fill in the blanks using the words given in parentheses.*

(delegation, nursing care plan, scope, nursing process)

1. The _____ _____ _____ is a specific plan of care for each patient or resident developed by the nursing team.

2. The _____ _____ is a process that allows members of the nursing team to communicate with each other regarding the patient's or resident's specific nursing care needs.

3. To ensure that the nursing team functions efficiently, an RN or LPN has the authority to assign selected tasks to a nursing assistant; this is also known as _____.

4. The range of tasks that a nursing assistant is legally permitted to do is called the _____ of practice.

LEGAL AND ETHICAL ASPECTS OF THE NURSING ASSISTANT'S JOB

Key Learning Points

- A Patient's Bill of Rights
- Resident's rights set by OBRA
- The seven civil law violations in the workplace (defamation, assault, battery, fraud, false imprisonment, invasion of privacy, and larceny)
- How to avoid the seven civil law violations in the workplace
- Forms of abuse
- Reporting abuse
- Ethical standards that govern the nursing profession
- The words *laws, civil laws, criminal laws, tort, unintentional tort, negligent, malpractice, intentional tort, slander, libel, informed consent, confidentiality, HIPAA, abuse, ethics,* and *value*

Activity A *Mark each statement as either "true" (T) or "false" (F). Correct the false statements.*

1. T F A patient cannot suggest alternatives to his or her planned care, or transfer to another facility if he or she so desires.

2. T F A patient must have information about his or her diagnosis, treatment, and prognosis.

3. T F All communication (written and oral) related to a patient's care need not be treated with confidentiality.

4. T F A patient can participate in, or decline to participate in, experimental studies.

5. T F   A patient has a right to receive considerate and respectful care.

Activity B *Place an "X" next to statements that are part of the Resident Rights.*

1. _____ A resident cannot share a room with a spouse if both partners are residents in the same facility.

2. _____ A resident can control his or her own finances.

3. _____ A resident cannot have information about the facility's compliance with regulations.

4. _____ A resident can have privacy—including privacy while receiving treatments and nursing care, making and receiving telephone calls, sending and receiving mail, and receiving visitors—and have personal and medical records treated confidentially.

5. _____ A resident can have information about eligibility for Medicare or Medicaid funds and be protected against Medicaid discrimination.

Activity C *Match the civil law violations, given in Column A, with their descriptions, given in Column B.*

Column A	Column B
_____ 1. Defamation	a. Violating a person's right to confidentiality
_____ 2. Assault	b. Touching a person without the person's informed consent
_____ 3. Battery	
_____ 4. Fraud	c. Stealing another person's property
_____ 5. False imprisonment	d. Hurting another person's reputation by making untrue statements
_____ 6. Invasion of privacy	e. Causing harm to another person by deception
_____ 7. Larceny	f. Confining another person against his or her will
	g. Causing a person to fear bodily harm by threatening or attempting to touch a person without his consent

Activity D *Select the single best answer for each of the following questions.*

1. Striking, biting, slapping, shaking, and handling another person roughly are all actions that make up:
   a. Emotional abuse
   b. Physical abuse
   c. Psychological abuse
   d. Involuntary seclusion

2. Making another person fearful by threatening him or her with physical harm, teasing a person in a cruel way, and abandonment are forms of:
   a. Physical abuse
   b. Sexual abuse
   c. Slander
   d. Psychological abuse

3. Making inappropriate, sexually aggressive comments, and threatening or forcing another person to engage in sexual activity are forms of:
   a. Assault
   b. Negligence
   c. Sexual abuse
   d. Involuntary seclusion

> Abuse is a criminal act and is punishable by a court of law.

Activity E *Select the single best answer to the following question.*

1. What should you do when you suspect that one of your patients or residents is being abused?
   a. Report suspicions to the proper person in the facility.
   b. Investigate whether abuse has actually occurred.
   c. Investigate who has caused the abuse.
   d. Ignore it and don't get involved.

Activity F *Place an "X" next to the actions that do NOT conform to the ethical standards of the nursing profession.*

1. _____ Treat patients and residents with respect for their individual needs and values.

2. ____ Do not allow the patient or resident to control his or her own care.

3. ____ Pass on information about patients and residents learned in the health care setting to his or her family and friends.

4. ____ Be guided by consideration for the dignity of patients and residents.

5. ____ Fulfill the obligation to provide competent care to patients and residents.

Activity G *Fill in the blanks using the words given in parentheses.*

(federal privacy, intentional, unintentional, confidentiality, informed consent)

1. A/an _____ tort occurs when someone causes harm or injury to another person or that person's property by accident.

2. A violation of civil law committed by a person with the intent to do harm is considered a/an _____ tort.

3. Permission granted by a patient or resident to begin treatment or perform a procedure after receiving a full explanation of the treatment or procedure from the health care provider is called _____.

4. Keeping personal information that someone shares with you to yourself is called _____.

5. Health Insurance Portability and Accountability Act (HIPAA) is a/an _____ _____ regulation that helps to keep personal information about patients and residents private.

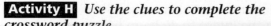

Activity H *Use the clues to complete the crossword puzzle.*

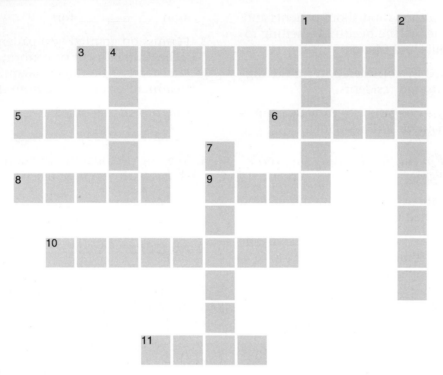

ACROSS

3. Negligence committed by people who hold licenses to practice their profession
5. A cherished belief or principle
6. Type of law concerned with relationships between individuals
8. Written statements that injure someone's reputation
9. Rules made by a governing authority with the intent of preserving basic human rights
10. Type of law concerned with the relationship between individual and society
11. Violation of civil law

DOWN

1. Moral principles or standards that govern conduct
2. A person who commits an unintentional tort
4. The repetitive and deliberate infliction of injury on another person
7. Spoken statements that injure someone's reputation

Professionalism and Job-Seeking Skills

WORKING AS A PROFESSIONAL

Key Learning Points

- Characteristics contributing to a strong work ethic
- Characteristics of a professional health care worker
- Guidelines to maintain a good physical and emotional health as a professional
- The words *professional, work ethic, hygiene,* and *attitude*

Activity A *Fill in the blanks using the words given in parentheses.*

(hygiene, work ethic, professional, attitude)

1. _____ A person who has credentials obtained through education and training that enables him or her to become licensed or certified to practice a certain profession; also, a person who demonstrates a professional attitude

2. _____ The side of ourselves that we display to the world, communicating outwardly how we feel about things

3. _____ Personal cleanliness

4. _____ A person's attitude toward his or her work

Activity B *Match the qualities of a professional, given in Column A, with the examples of them, given in Column B.*

Column A

_____ 1. Punctuality

_____ 2. Reliability

_____ 3. Accountability

_____ 4. Conscientious-ness

_____ 5. Courtesy and respectfulness

_____ 6. Honesty

_____ 7. Cooperative-ness

_____ 8. Empathy

Column B

a. You tell the truth and do not lie, cheat, or steal.

b. You are polite and do not make negative remarks about your coworkers.

c. Your supervisor can depend on you to finish your assignment properly.

d. You offer a helping hand when you see that a coworker requires help.

e. You take responsibility for your actions and their consequences.

f. You are always on time for work.

g. You are able to show kindness and tolerance by imagining yourself in someone else's situation.

h. You take your work seriously and ask for clarification or help when you need it.

Activity C *To maintain good physical health, a nursing assistant must take care of himself or herself first. Look at the figures below and fill in the blanks.*

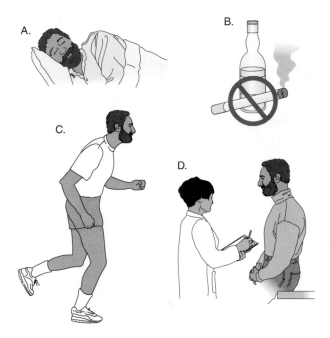

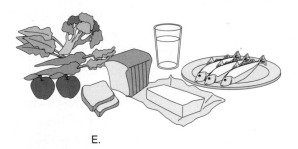

A. You should get enough s _____ .

B. You should not s _____ and you should limit your a _____ intake.

C. You should e _____ regularly.

D. You should have a routine p _____
e _____ .

E. You should eat w _____ -b _____
meals.

Activity D *Select the single best answer for each of the following questions.*

1. Why is it important for a nursing assistant to maintain good personal hygiene?

  a. Good personal hygiene helps to prevent the spread of infection.

  b. Good personal hygiene sets you apart from other nursing assistants.

  c. Good personal hygiene makes you eligible for a raise in salary.

  d. Good personal hygiene sets an example for your patients and residents.

2. Which of the following activities is NOT a part of maintaining good personal hygiene?

  a. Bathing daily and using a deodorant

  b. Keeping your nails short and clean

  c. Wearing a clean, pressed uniform everyday

  d. Wearing jewelry to improve your appearance

Activity E *Mark each statement as either "true" (T) or "false" (F). Correct the false statements.*

1. T F Physical activity relieves mental and emotional stress.

2. T F Making time for yourself will not help you when you feel overwhelmed with responsibilities.

3. T F You must never ask to be assigned to different work areas or to different patients or residents.

Activity F *Select the single best answer for each of the following questions.*

1. A strong "work ethic" is one of the most important qualities that potential employers look for in a nursing assistant. What does this term refer to?

  a. A person's ability to judge whether a nurse has made a correct decision

  b. A person's ability to perform the work assigned to him or her

c. A person's attitude toward his or her work

d. A person's awareness of the rules that should be followed in the workplace

2. Which of the following qualities does NOT reflect a strong work ethic?

a. Punctuality

b. Competitiveness

c. Accountability

d. Reliability

FINDING A JOB

Key Learning Points

■ Considerations before beginning a job search
■ Places to search for job openings
■ Completing a job application
■ Making a good first impression during an interview
■ The words *resume, reference list,* and *interview*

Activity A *Match the characteristics of a nursing assistant, given in Column A, with the health care facility that he or she would be best suited for, given in Column B.*

Column A	Column B
_____ **1.** Likes to work with elderly people	**a.** Hospice organization
_____ **2.** Wants to care for people in their homes	**b.** Long-term care facility
_____ **3.** Wants to provide comfort to dying people and their families	**c.** Home health care agency

Activity B *Sally is searching for a suitable nursing assistant job. Considering her situation, help her make a decision from the given options. Select the single best answer for each of the following situations.*

Sally has a child.

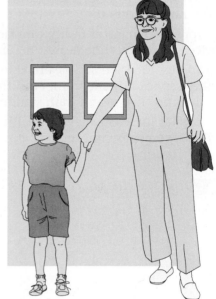

a. She takes the child to work.

b. She works whatever shift she is scheduled for, not considering the childcare arrangements.

c. She tells the employer that she is available to work any shift, even though this is not true.

d. She tells the employer what shift she is available to work, based on her childcare arrangements.

Sally plans to take the bus to get to work.

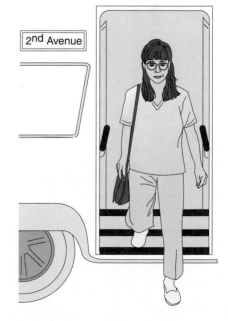

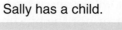

a. She applies for a job at every health care facility, whether or not the bus line nearest to her home serves it.

b. She applies for a job at health care facilities serviced by the bus line nearest her home.

c. She applies for a job at a health care facility serviced by the train, even though she does not live near a train station.

d. She applies for a job at every health care facility, even those not served by public transportation.

Activity C *Use the clues to complete the crossword puzzle.*

ACROSS

2. Check here for a list of facilities and agencies that hire nursing assistants
4. Contains classified ads listing employment opportunities
5. They may know of possible job openings
6. Many schools and facilities have one of these, where job opportunities may be posted

DOWN

1. A department at your school that may have job listings and can often help with writing a résumé
3. Web sites that help people find jobs are located here

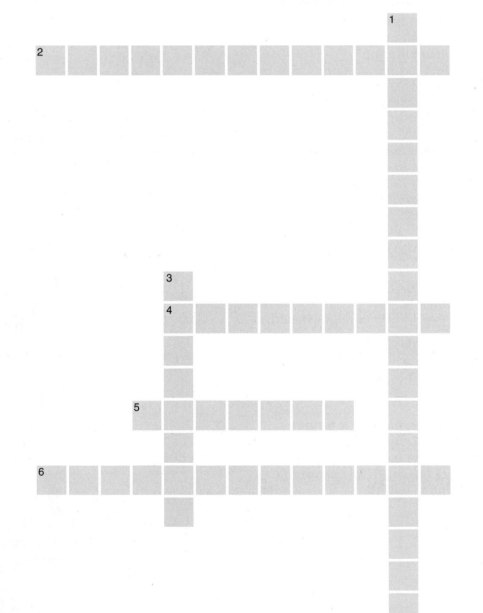

Note: Advance planning about the type of employment you want helps to give your job search direction.

Activity D *Match the words, given in Column A, with their meanings, given in Column B.*

Column A

_____ **1.** Résumé

_____ **2.** Cover letter

_____ **3.** Reference list

_____ **4.** Interview

Column B

a. A meeting between an employer and a potential employee, during which information is exchanged regarding the organization, the job, and the potential employee's qualifications for the job

b. A list of three or four people willing to talk to a potential employer about your abilities

c. A brief document that gives general information about you, your education, and work experience to a potential employer

d. A letter to introduce yourself to a potential employer

Activity E *Place an "X" next to the information that should be included in a résumé.*

1. _____ Full name

2. _____ Employment history

3. _____ Weight

4. _____ Marital status

5. _____ Age

6. _____ Address

7. _____ Education history

8. _____ Sexual preference

Activity F *Think About It! Briefly* [answer] *the following question in the space provided.*

Amy Robinson goes on an interview for a position as a nursing assistant at a long-term care facility. The interviewer asks Amy whether or not she is married. How should Amy respond to the interviewer's question?

_____

_____

Activity G

Which one of the nursing assistants pictured below is most likely to make a favorable impression on a potential employer?

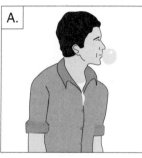
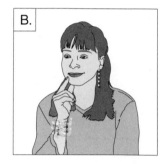
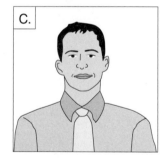
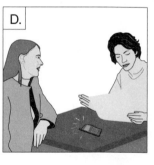

CHAPTER 4

Communication Skills

INTRODUCTION TO COMMUNICATION

Key Learning Points

- Importance of communicating effectively
- Two major forms of communication
- Techniques that promote effective communication
- The words *communication, verbal communication,* and *nonverbal communication*

Activity A *Communication is the exchange of information. Conversation is a form of communication. Look at the following picture and fill in the blanks using the words in parentheses. (You may use some words more than once.)*

(message, sender, feedback, receiver)

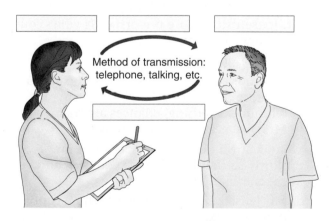

Method of transmission: telephone, talking, etc.

The _____ is the person with information to share, and the _____ is the person for whom the information is intended. The _____ delivers the information in the form of a _____, which the receiver may or may not understand. Through _____, or a return message, the _____ lets the _____ know whether the message was received and understood.

Activity B *Select the single best answer for each of the following questions.*

1. Which of the following activities is a form of communication?
   a. Telling someone something
   b. Giving a gift to someone
   c. Accepting a gift from someone
   d. Driving down to a friend's house to meet him

2. Which of the following is an example of verbal communication?
   a. Unintentional facial expressions
   b. Shaking the hand of a new patient or resident
   c. Writing out a question to a deaf resident
   d. Body language

3. Which of the following statements indicates that Mrs. Smith is using a form of nonverbal communication?
   a. Mrs. Smith walks over to the room next to hers to talk to another resident.
   b. Mrs. Smith grimaces and groans softly when she gets up from her bed and attempts to stand.

c. Mrs. Smith talks about a pain in her back to a nursing assistant.

d. Mrs. Smith listens carefully to the doctor who is informing her about her condition.

Activity C *Place a "V" next to the statements that are examples of verbal communication, and an "N" next to the statements that are examples of nonverbal communication.*

1. _____ Use of language, either spoken or written

2. _____ Gently touching a patient or a resident on the shoulder to reassure her

3. _____ Making a face when you put weight on a painful leg

4. _____ Making a telephone call

5. _____ Nodding as someone speaks

6. _____ Tapping your fingers on the table because you are bored

7. _____ Recording vital sign measurements in a patient's or resident's chart

Nursing assistants are an important link between the patient or resident and other members of the health care team. The nursing assistant is often the first member of the health care team to become aware of a change in a patient's or resident's condition that could be a sign of something serious. This is why it is important for nursing assistants to have good communication skills.

Activity D *Fill in the blanks using the words given in parentheses.*

(nonverbal communication, communication, verbal communication)

1. The exchange of information is known

   as _____.

2. Communicating with facial expressions, gestures, and body language, instead of written or spoken language, is

   called _____.

3. Communication in written or spoken

   language is known as _____.

Activity E *List three reasons why it is important for a nursing assistant to be a successful communicator.*

_____

_____

_____

Note: Listening is one of the most important communication skills, especially in the health care field.

COMMUNICATING WITH PEOPLE WITH SPECIAL NEEDS

Key Learning Points

- Situations that might affect a person's ability to communicate effectively
- Assisting with communication in these situations

Activity A *List three situations that may affect a person's ability to communicate effectively.*

_____

_____

_____

Activity B *Select the single best answer for the following question.*

1. Mr. Jensen is 85 years old and has a hearing problem due to old age. What would be the best form of communicating with Mr. Jensen so that he understands what you are trying to tell him?

   a. Speak as loudly as you can.

   b. Get your coworker to help you in communicating. When two people are trying to tell him something, chances are that Mr. Jensen will get the message.

   c. Look at Mr. Jensen and speak to him slowly so that he can read your lips and get the message.

   d. Mr. Jensen is a very old man. There is no point in talking to him.

Activity C *Place an "X" next to the proper ways to communicate with a person who is hearing impaired.*

1. _____ Face the person while talking to him.

2. _____ Use sign language.

3. _____ Use a note pad and write down important questions or directions.

Activity D *List three guidelines for communicating effectively with a person who has a speech difficulty.*

_____

_____

_____

RESOLVING CONFLICTS

Key Learning Points

- The word *conflict*
- Causes of conflict and ways of resolving it

Activity A *There are different ways to resolve a conflict. Place a "T" next to the sentences that describe an effective way of resolving a conflict and an "F" next to the sentences that describe ineffective ways of resolving a conflict. Correct the statements that you marked "F".*

1. _____ Arrange to speak privately with the person you have a conflict with.

2. _____ Ask a supervisor to mediate immediately.

3. _____ During the conversation, focus on the area of conflict.

4. _____ Be specific about what you understand the problem to be.

5. _____ Tell the person how you feel about him or her.

6. _____ Say, "You really hurt my feelings by what you said the other day."

7. _____ Agree to disagree.

8. _____ Offer advice to the person.

Activity B *Select the single best answer for the following question.*

1. Conflict between people can occur when one person:
   a. Is unable to understand or accept another's ideas or beliefs
   b. Has expectations that differ from those of the other person
   c. Misunderstands another person's words or intentions
   d. All of the above

Activity C *Define the word* conflict.

_____

_____

_____

USING THE TELEPHONE

Key Learning Points

- Proper telephone communication skills
- Information that a nursing assistant is not permitted to communicate via the telephone

Activity A *Select the single best answer for the following question.*

1. As a nursing assistant, you are responsible for answering the telephone, either at the nursing station or in a patient's or resident's room. When answering the telephone, what should you NOT do?
   a. Speak in a pleasant and unhurried voice
   b. Take a message by writing down the caller's name and telephone number and delivering the message to the person it is intended for
   c. Convey a kind and professional attitude
   d. Provide information about a patient's or resident's condition to the caller

Activity B *Place an "X" next to the incorrect statements.*

1. _____ Answer the phone promptly within the first three rings.

2. _____ Start by asking the caller about the information he or she wants.

3. _____ Identify yourself by name, by title, and by your unit or floor according to the facility policy.

4. _____ Ask "How may I help you?" since the caller has called to gather information.

5. _____ Know how to perform basic functions using your facilities telephone system, such as transferring a call or placing a caller on hold.

6. _____ Put the caller on hold if you have more pressing tasks to attend to.

7. _____ Do not take any message from the caller. It is not part of a nursing assistant's duty.

8. _____ Doctors' orders and diagnostic test results can be given to a nursing assistant over the telephone.

9. _____ Do not use the telephone at the nurse's station to make or receive personal calls.

COMMUNICATION AMONG MEMBERS OF THE HEALTH CARE TEAM

Key Learning Points

- Why a nursing assistant is often considered the "eyes and ears" of the health care team
- Methods of reporting and recording information in a health care setting
- The words *observations, objective data, signs, subjective data, symptom, reporting, recording, medical record (chart),* and *Kardex*

Activity A *Select the single best answer for the following question.*

1. Which of the following is subjective data?

    a. Mrs. Smith's complaint of abdominal pain immediately after a meal

    b. Mrs. Smith's temperature

    c. Mrs. Smith's urine output

    d. Mrs. Smith's pulse rate

Activity B *Define the words* reporting *and* recording.

_____

_____

_____

_____

Activity C *List the guidelines that nursing assistants need to follow while recording.*

_____

_____

_____

_____

_____

_____

_____

_____

_____

Activity D *Fill in the blanks using the words given in parentheses.*

(Kardex, signs, observation, symptoms, subjective data, objective data, medical record)

1. Something that you notice about a patient or resident, typically related to a change in the person's physical or mental

    condition, is a/an _____.

2. Objective evidence of disease, observations based on data that is obtained directly, through measurements, or by using one of the five senses, are called

_____.

3. Subjective evidence of disease based on data that cannot be measured or observed first-hand, such as a patient's or resident's complaint of pain, are called

_____.

4. A card file that contains versions of each patient's or resident's medical record is a

_____.

5. A legal document, also called a medical chart, where information about a patient's or resident's current condition, the measures that have been taken by the medical or nursing staff to diagnose and treat the condition, and the patient's or resident's response to the treatment and care provided is recorded is a _____ _____.

6. Information that is obtained directly, through measurements, or by using one of the five senses (sight, smell, taste, hearing, touch) is called

_____ _____.

7. Information that cannot be objectively measured or assessed is called

_____ _____.

Activity E *Explain why a nursing assistant is considered the "eyes and ears" of the health care team.*

_____
_____
_____
_____
_____
_____
_____

CHAPTER 5

Those We Care For

GROWTH AND DEVELOPMENT

Key Learning Points

- Stages of human growth and development
- The words *growth*, *development*, and *tasks*

Activity A *Match the stages of growth and development, given in Column A, with their characteristics, given in Column B.*

Column A	Column B
_____ 1. Infancy	a. A stage of gender identity
_____ 2. Toddlerhood	b. A stage of active imagination
_____ 3. Preschool	c. A stage of sharing wisdom but failing health
_____ 4. School-age	d. A stage of toilet training
_____ 5. Adolescence	e. A stage of assuming a caretaker's role
_____ 6. Middle adulthood	f. A stage of rapid physical and psychological growth
_____ 7. Older adulthood	g. A stage of questioning authority

Activity B *Select the single best answer for each of the following questions.*

1. From the following examples of changes that can occur in the human body, which one is an example of "growth"?
   a. Changes in the height and weight of a person
   b. Changes in the behavior of a person
   c. Changes in the way a person thinks
   d. Changes in the way a person interacts socially

2. Which of the following is typical of the process of "development"?
   a. Changes in a person's height and weight
   b. Changes in a person's bank account
   c. Changes in a person's behavior and way of thinking
   d. Changes in a person's sexual preferences

3. Which of the following is true of the "tasks" that a person must complete?
   a. A person cannot progress to the next stage of development without successfully completing them.
   b. A person can progress to the next stage of development without successfully completing them.
   c. A person can jump directly to the next stage of development.
   d. A person can constantly switch between different stages of development.

BASIC HUMAN NEEDS

Key Learning Points

- Each level of Maslow's hierarchy of basic human needs
- Ways that a nursing assistant helps patients and residents to meet their needs
- The word *needs*

Activity A *Maslow's pyramid identifies the hierarchy of human needs. In the following figure, write down the correct order of needs from the list A.–E. below. Then give an example of a way that a nursing assistant may be able to help a patient or resident meet each level of these needs.*

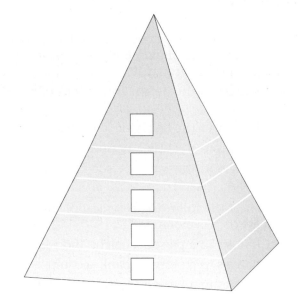

A. Self-esteem needs _____

_____

_____

B. Physiological needs _____

_____

_____

C. Safety and security needs _____

_____

_____

D. Self-actualization needs _____ _____

_____

_____

E. Love and belonging needs _____

_____

_____

Activity B *Select the single best answer for each of the following questions.*

1. When a nursing assistant assists a patient or resident with toileting, which of Maslow's needs does the nursing assistant help the person to meet?
   a. Love and belonging need
   b. Self-esteem need
   c. Self-actualization need
   d. Physiological need

2. Which of the following actions help to fulfill a patient's or resident's need for love and belonging?
   a. A gentle touch
   b. Making sure the wheels of the wheelchair are locked
   c. Helping the patient or resident set realistic goals
   d. Assisting the patient or resident with basic grooming

3. Which of the following is not a physical need?
   a. Shelter
   b. Food
   c. Acceptance
   d. Air

4. Which of the following is not a basic human need?
   a. Safety and security
   b. Self-esteem
   c. Self-actualization
   d. Fear

5. Which of the following is essential to a person's physical and mental health?
   a. Task
   b. Desire
   c. Need
   d. Demand

HUMAN SEXUALITY AND INTIMACY

Key Learning Points

- Difference between sex and sexuality
- Ways in which nursing assistants can help patients and residents to fulfill their need to be thought of as sexual beings
- The words *sexuality, intimacy, sex,* and *masturbation*

Activity A *Select the single best answer for each of the following questions.*

1. A resident in a long-term care facility expresses a desire to have a sexual relationship with you. What would you do?
   a. Ignore the resident.
   b. Complain to the nurse.
   c. Giggle and tease the resident in a flirtatious manner.
   d. Tell the resident kindly, yet firmly, that you are not going to do what he or she is asking you to do.

2. Which of the following conditions may affect the person's feelings about his or her sexuality?
   a. Mrs. Robinson has to have surgery for the removal of a cancerous breast.
   b. Mr. Smith's gangrenous right leg has to be amputated.
   c. Mrs. Ching's face is burned.
   d. All of the above

Activity B *Think About It! Briefly answer the following question in the space provided.*

What would you do if you saw a resident masturbating in a public room?

_____

_____

_____

Activity C *Fill in the blanks using the words given in parentheses.*

(sex, intimacy, sexuality, masturbation)

a. When human beings feel close to others and share an emotional rapport with them, they are said to share _____ with them.

b. Self-stimulation of the genitals for sexual pleasure or release is called _____.

c. _____ is the physical activity one engages in to obtain sexual pleasure and reproduce.

d. _____ is how a person perceives his or her maleness or femaleness.

CULTURE AND RELIGION

Key Learning Points

- The effect of culture and religion on how a person views illness and health care
- Importance of health care workers recognizing their patients' and residents' cultural and religious differences
- The words *culture, race,* and *religion*

Activity A *Place a "C" next to the statements that are related to a person's culture, an "RE" next to the statements that are related to a person's religion, and an "RA" next to the statements that are related to a person's race.*

1. _____ A person of African descent has dark skin and curly, black hair.

2. _____ A Jewish person does not want to have his long beard shaved.

3. _____ An Asian person has great respect for his elders.

4. _____ A Middle Eastern woman is not allowed to be questioned or examined by a male health care provider unless her husband is present.

5. _____ An Asian person has almond-shaped eyes and straight black hair.

6. _____ A person from Panama believes that wearing strings on the wrist will relieve pain.

7. _____ A Catholic person does not want to eat meat on Fridays during Lent.

Activity B *Mark each statement as either "true" (T) or "false" (F). Correct the false statements.*

1. **T F**   An Islamic patient refuses to shave his beard. The health care provider should consider this as a silly whim.

2. **T F**   A Japanese resident prefers freshly cooked rice to loaves of bread. The health care provider should understand his dietary habits and not force him to switch to bread.

3. **T F**   A female patient who is a Pagan does not want to attend a lecture delivered by the local priest. The health care provider should ask her to change her anti-Christian views on things.

Activity C *Fill in the blanks using the words given in parentheses.*

(religion, culture, race)

a. _____ is a general characterization that describes skin color, body stature, facial features, and hair texture.

b. _____ defines a person's spiritual beliefs.

c. The beliefs, values, and traditions that are customary to a group of people are defined

   by the term _____.

QUALITY OF LIFE

Key Learning Points

- The concept of "quality of life"
- The importance of health care workers in respecting patients' and residents' decisions regarding their own quality of life

Activity A *Fill in the blanks using the words given in parentheses.*

1. A _____ (simplistic/holistic) approach to health care takes into consideration a person's emotional needs as well as his or her physical ones.

2. The idea of what quality of life means is

   _____ (different/similar) for each person and may change as a person's situation changes.

Activity B *Think About It! Briefly answer the following question in the space provided.*

Mr. Pyne was treated for heart problems a few months ago. He continues to smoke heavily, despite his heart problems. He also won't eat anything but steak, and he rarely exercises. The first time that he was hospitalized for his heart problems, the health care team advised Mr. Pyne to stop smoking and to begin eating a heart-healthy diet and exercising, but he seems not to have taken that advice. Now Mr. Pyne is back in the hospital again. If you were a member of the health care team who cared for Mr. Pyne the first time, how would you feel toward him now?

_____

_____

_____

WHAT IS IT LIKE TO BE A PATIENT OR RESIDENT?

Key Learning Points

- How being a patient or resident can affect how a person acts toward others
- How it would feel to be a patient or resident

Activity A *Think About It! Briefly answer the following question in the space provided.*

Mr. Simon is a resident at the health care facility where you work. He has severe arthritis, and his children live far away and rarely come to visit. He is very critical and rarely has anything pleasant to say to you or to anyone else. Why might Mr. Simon be acting this way?

_____

_____

_____

_____

_____

_____

CHAPTER 6

The Patient's or Resident's Environment

THE PHYSICAL ENVIRONMENT

Key Learning Points

- Aspects of the physical environment that affect safety and comfort
- Role in helping to keep the patient's or resident's environment clean, comfortable, and safe
- The Omnibus Budget Reconciliation Act (OBRA) regulations relating to the physical environment in long-term care facilities

Activity A *To ensure the safety and comfort of patients and residents, standards are set that help regulate the physical environment. Mark each statement as either "true" (T) or "false" (F). Correct the false statements.*

1. **T F** Cleanliness is essential for controlling the spread of infection.

2. **T F** The AHA sets the standards for the residents' environment in a long-term care facility.

3. **T F** People who are ill or elderly prefer a cooler room temperature.

4. **T F** The use of facility-approved air fresheners helps to control odors.

Activity B *Nursing assistants perform many tasks to help ensure cleanliness and a good quality of life for the people they care for. Mark each statement as either "true" (T) or "false" (F). Correct the false statements.*

1. **T F** Each member of the health care team is responsible for keeping the facility clean.

2. **T F** A nursing assistant does major, routine cleaning of the facility.

3. **T F** The custodial staff is responsible for changing the bed linens according to facility policy.

4. **T F** A nursing assistant helps to keep the personal belongings of the patient or resident neat and clean.

5. **T F** If you notice something spilled on the floor or a countertop, you should call for the housekeeping staff immediately.

6. **T F** If you see a stray piece of trash, you should pick it up and dispose of it properly.

7. **T F** If you notice that there is an ongoing problem, such as wastebaskets not being emptied or bathrooms not being cleaned properly, you should report this observation to the housekeeping department, so that they can follow up with the appropriate people.

Activity C *As a nursing assistant, what would you do to control odor and maintain a pleasant environment in the given situations?*

1. A resident is sick with stomach flu and vomits frequently.

   _____

2. A resident is incontinent of urine.

   _____

3. A resident uses the bedpan to have a bowel movement and is embarrassed by the odor.

   _____

4. A resident who is incontinent of feces must wear disposable briefs.

   _____

Activity D *Select the single best answer for each of the following questions.*

1. You are working in a long-term care facility. While moving around, you feel too warm but your patient or resident is comfortable. What would you do in these circumstances?

   a. Switch on a fan

   b. Turn up the air conditioning

   c. Open a window

   d. Plan for the warmer temperatures and dress accordingly

2. Which of the following will help decrease unnecessary noise in a hospital or a health care facility?

   a. Answering the phones promptly

   b. Reporting noisy equipment that needs to be oiled

   c. Being aware of the volume of your own voice

   d. All of the above

3. Which of the following types of lighting helps to prevent eye strain while reading?

   a. Task lighting

   b. General lighting

   c. Sunlight

   d. A night light

FURNITURE AND EQUIPMENT

Key Learning Points

- The standard equipment and furniture found in a person's room in a health care facility
- Changing the height and mattress position of an adjustable bed
- Importance of allowing a person to have and display personal items
- Defining the words *unit* and *gatch*

Activity A *Write the names next to the description of the furniture or objects that are typically found in a patient's or resident's unit, as shown in each figure below.*

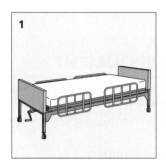

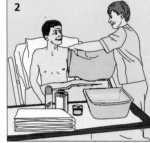

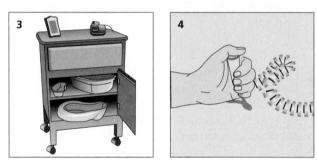

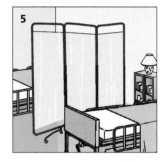

1. Has unique features such as wheels, side rails, and controls for adjusting bed height and the position of the mattress

   _____

2. Fits over a bed or chair and is used as a work surface _____

3. Storage unit for personal care items and equipment _____

4. Used to communicate with the health care staff _____

5. Used to protect the patient's or resident's modesty when providing care

   _____

Activity B *Think About It! Briefly answer the following question in the space provided.*

Adjustable beds have several features that regular beds do not have: controls for adjusting the height of the bed and the position of the mattress, wheels, and side rails. Explain the purpose of each of these special features. Also explain when to lock the wheels on the bed, and why it is important to remember to do this.

_____

_____

_____

_____

_____

_____

_____

Activity C *Fill in the blanks using the words given in parentheses.*

(Fowler's position, Trendelenburg's position, reverse Trendelenburg's position)

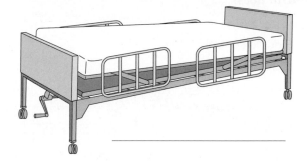

_____

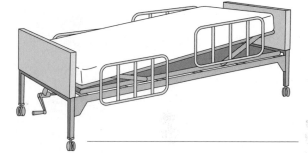

_____

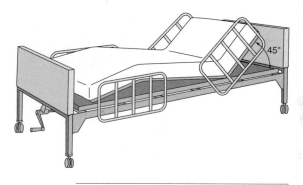

_____

Activity D *Many of the beds used in health care settings have controls for adjusting the bed height and the position of the mattress. These controls can be electric or manual. Look at the pictures below and write down what each control does.*

A. Electric controls

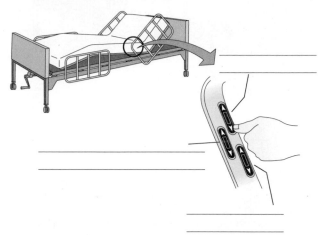

_____

_____

_____

B. Manual controls

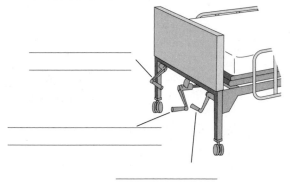

_____

_____

_____

_____

_____

_____

Activity E *State the importance of allowing a person to have and display his or her personal items in the health care facility.*

_____

_____

_____

_____

_____

_____

Activity F *Fill in the blanks using the words given in parentheses.*

(unit, gatch)

1. The joint at the hips and knees of the mattresses of most adjustable beds, which allows the mattresses to "break" so that the person's head can be elevated and his or her knees can be bent, is called a _____

2. A patient's or resident's room is also called a

_____

CHAPTER 7

Basic Body Structure and Function

HOW IS THE BODY ORGANIZED?

Key Learning Points

- The basic organizational levels of the body
- The words *cell, tissue, organ, organ system, nutrients, metabolism,* and *homeostasis*

Activity A *All living things share the same basic levels of organization. Look at the following figure. Fill in the boxes below with the correct order of the levels of organization.*

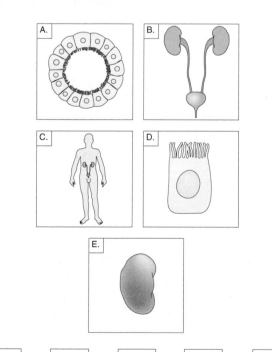

Activity B *Match the words, given in Column A, with their description, given in Column B.*

Column A

_____ **1.** Cell

_____ **2.** Tissue

_____ **3.** Organ

_____ **4.** Organ system

_____ **5.** Nutrients

_____ **6.** Metabolism

_____ **7.** Homeostasis

Column B

a. Substances in food and fluids that the body uses to grow

b. A state of balance

c. The basic unit of life

d. The physical and chemical changes that occur when the cells of the body change the food that we eat into energy

e. A group of cells similar in structure, and specialized to perform a specific function

f. A group of tissues functioning together for a similar purpose

g. A group of organs working together to perform a specific function for the body

THE INTEGUMENTARY SYSTEM

Key Learning Points

- Main parts of the integumentary system
- Major functions of the integumentary system
- Layers of the skin
- Normal changes in the integumentary system due to aging
- The words *epidermis, dermis, melanin, subcutaneous tissue,* and *sebum*

Activity A *Place an "X" next to the parts of the body listed below that are a part of the integumentary system.*

1. _____ Skin

2. _____ Kidneys

3. _____ Hair

4. _____ Eye

5. _____ Nails

6. _____ Sweat glands

7. _____ Sebaceous glands

Activity B *Mark each statement as either "true" (T) or "false" (F). Correct the false statements.*

1. T F   The integumentary system helps to maintain the body's homeostasis.

2. T F   The integumentary system regulates the temperature of the body.

3. T F   The skin is the body's largest organ.

4. T F   Nails are made of special skin cells that have been hardened by a protein called melanin.

Activity C *The figure shows a cross-section of the skin. Label the figure using the words given in parentheses.*

(hair follicle, dermis, epidermis, melanin-producing cells, sweat gland, subcutaneous tissue)

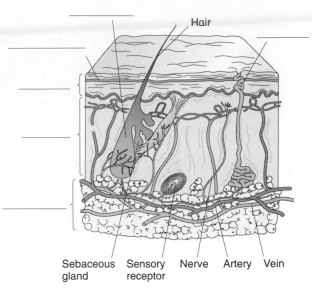

Hair

Sebaceous gland   Sensory receptor   Nerve   Artery   Vein

Activity D *Listed below are the effects of aging on the integumentary system. Fill in the blanks using the words given in parentheses.*

(melanin, skin, fragile, age spots, nails)

1. The skin becomes thin, _____, and dry, putting the person at risk for skin injury.

2. The _____ become thick, tough, and yellow.

3. Loss of _____ causes the hair to turn gray.

4. Deposits of melanin in certain areas, such as the backs of the hands and the face, lead to the formation of _____.

5. Blood flow to the _____ decreases, resulting in slower healing if injury occurs.

Activity E *Match the words, given in Column A, with their descriptions, given in Column B.*

Column A	Column B
_____ 1. Epidermis	a. An oily substance secreted by glands in the skin that lubricates the skin and helps to prevent it from drying out
_____ 2. Dermis	
_____ 3. Melanin	
_____ 4. Subcutaneous tissue	
_____ 5. Sebum	b. A dark pigment that gives our skin, hair, and eyes color

c. The outer layer of the skin

d. The deepest layer of the skin, where sensory receptors, blood vessels, nerves, glands, and hair follicles are found

e. The layer of fat that supports the dermis

THE MUSCULOSKELETAL SYSTEM

Key Learning Points

- Main parts of the musculoskeletal system
- Main functions of the musculoskeletal system
- The four general types of bones
- The three general types of joints
- Normal changes in the musculoskeletal system due to aging
- The words *skeleton, joint, cartilage, ligaments, tendons,* and *atrophy*

Activity A *Place an "X" next to the parts of the body listed below that are a part of the musculoskeletal system.*

1. ____ Skin
2. ____ Bones
3. ____ Blood
4. ____ Joints
5. ____ Muscles

Activity B *Mark each statement as either "true" (T) or "false" (F). Correct the false statements.*

1. T F Sodium, an important mineral that keeps the bones strong and helps the cardiac muscle to function properly, is stored in the bones.

2. T F Contraction of the muscles helps us to maintain an upright posture.

3. T F Contraction of the skeletal muscles helps us to maintain a constant body temperature by cooling us down.

4. T F Contracting a muscle causes it to shorten, resulting in movement.

5. T F Blood cells are made in the bone marrow.

Activity C *Fill in the blanks using the words given in parentheses.*

(flat, face, long, shaft, short, thin, irregular)

1. _____ bones are found in the arms and the legs.

2. Flat bones are relatively _____ and may be curved.

3. Irregular bones are found in the spinal column and _____.

4. _____ bones are round or cube-shaped.

5. Long bones have a _____ and two rounded ends.

6. Oddly shaped bones that are not flat are called _____ bones.

7. The bones that form the skull are

_____.

Activity D *Match the classification of joints, given in Column A, with their location, given in Column B.*

Column A

____ 1. Fixed joints
____ 2. Slightly movable joints
____ 3. Freely movable joints

Column B

a. The spine
b. The fingers
c. The skull

Activity E *Think About It! Briefly answer the following question in the space provided.*

The normal process of aging causes significant changes in the musculoskeletal system. List three normal age-related changes that affect the musculoskeletal system. Then describe how each of these changes can affect the elderly people under your care, especially if other factors are present that make these changes occur at a much faster rate.

1. _____

_____

2. _____

_____

3. _____

_____

Activity F *Use the clues to complete the crossword puzzle.*

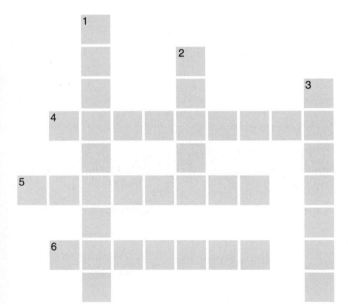

ACROSS

4. This acts as a "shock absorber"
5. The framework for the body formed by the bones
6. The loss of muscle size and strength

DOWN

1. These attach one bone to another, stabilizing the joint
2. The area where two bones join together
3. Bands of connective tissue that attach the skeletal muscles to the bones

THE RESPIRATORY SYSTEM

Key Learning Points

- Main parts of the respiratory system
- Main functions of the respiratory system
- Normal changes that occur in the musculoskeletal system due to aging
- The words *mucous membrane, mucus, respiration, gas exchange,* and *diaphragm*

Activity A *A figure of the respiratory system is shown below. Label the figure using the words given in parentheses. Then, write each part next to its description in the list below.*

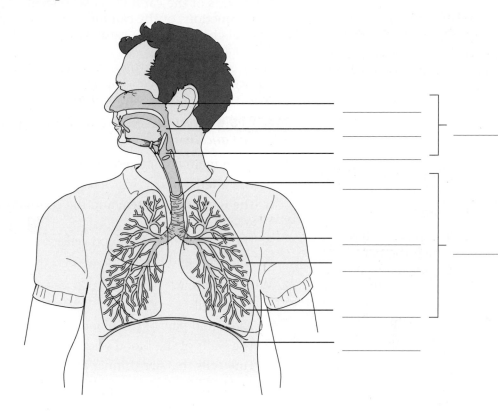

[pharynx, lower respiratory tract, larynx, bronchiole, bronchus, upper respiratory tract, diaphragm, lungs, trachea, nasal cavity]

1. The inside of the nose _____

2. The main organs of respiration _____

3. Connects each lung to the trachea _____

4. Strong muscle that separates the chest cavity from the abdominal cavity and assists in

   ventilation _____

5. Tiniest branches of the bronchi _____

6. Responsible for speech (also called the voice

   box) _____

7. Passage that carries air from the pharynx down into the chest toward the lungs (also

   called the windpipe) _____

8. The throat region _____

Activity B *Fill in the blanks using the words given in parentheses.*

(chemoreceptors, alveolus, intercostal muscles, inhalation, brain, diaphragm, exhalation)

1. Breathing has two phases: _____ and

   _____.

2. The _____ is a strong, dome-shaped muscle that separates the chest cavity from the abdominal cavity.

3. The _____ _____, which are located between the ribs, help with the respiratory effort.

4. The rate and depth of breathing is controlled

   mainly by the _____.

5. Special cells, called _____, located in the medulla and in some of the major arteries, monitor the amount of carbon dioxide and oxygen in the blood.

6. Carbon dioxide moves from the blood into the _____, and is removed from the body when we exhale.

Activity C *Think About It! Briefly answer the following question in the space provided.*

List two things you can do to help keep your respiratory system functioning properly well into old age.

1. _____

2. _____

Activity D *Match the words, given in Column A, with their descriptions, given in Column B.*

Column A

_____ **1.** Mucous membrane

_____ **2.** Mucus

_____ **3.** Respiration

_____ **4.** Gas exchange

_____ **5.** Diaphragm

Column B

a. The process during which the body obtains oxygen from the environment and removes carbon dioxide from the body

b. The strong, dome-shaped muscle that separates the chest cavity from the abdominal cavity and assists in breathing

c. A slippery, sticky substance that is secreted by special cells and serves to keep the surfaces of mucous membranes moist

d. A special type of epithelial tissue that lines many of the organ systems in the body and is coated with mucus

e. The transfer of oxygen into the blood, and carbon dioxide out of it

THE CARDIOVASCULAR SYSTEM

Key Learning Process

- Main parts of the cardiovascular system
- Main functions of the cardiovascular system
- Normal changes in the cardiovascular system due to aging
- The words *plasma, erythrocytes, hemoglobin, leukocytes, thrombocytes, circulation, cardiac cycle, systole, diastole,* and *varicose veins*

Activity A *Select the single best answer for the following questions.*

1. The two main components of blood are
   a. The arteries and veins
   b. The lymphatic system and the conduction system
   c. The plasma and the blood cells
   d. The heart and the heart valves

2. What is plasma?
   a. Blood cells
   b. The liquid part of the blood
   c. The walls of the blood vessels
   d. Tiny cells that are thinner at the edges

3. Why are the red blood cells red?
   a. Because hemoglobin turns bright red when combined with oxygen
   b. Because they are manufactured in the red bone marrow
   c. Because of the presence of plasma proteins
   d. Because lymph capillaries absorb fluid from the surrounding tissues

4. What is hemostasis?
   a. The process of allowing the blood vessels to constrict or dilate according to the body's needs
   b. The process that stops the flow of blood from the circulatory system by forming a clot
   c. The process of transferring substances in and out of the blood
   d. The process of returning the fluid that leaks into the tissues to the bloodstream

Activity B *Think About It! Briefly answer the following question in the space provided.*

List and describe two functions of the cardio-vascular system.

1. _____

2. _____

Activity C *Match the effects of aging on the cardiovascular system, given in Column A, with their descriptions, given in Column B.*

Column A

_____ 1. Less efficient heart contraction

_____ 2. Decreased elasticity in the arteries and veins

_____ 3. Decreased numbers of blood cells

Column B

a. The person feels dizzy or light headed when standing

b. Puts the person at a higher risk for developing infections

c. Tires faster while exercising

Activity D *Fill in the blanks using the words given in parentheses.*

(cardiac cycle, varicose veins, thrombocytes, plasma, systole, leukocytes, circulation, diastole, erythrocytes, hemoglobin)

1. The liquid part of blood is called

_____.

2. _____ are responsible for carrying oxygen to all the tissues of the body.

3. _____ is a protein found in red blood cells that combines with oxygen to carry it to the tissues of the body.

4. _____ are blood cells responsible for fighting infection.

5. Platelets or _____ are responsible for clotting of the blood.

6. The continuous movement of the blood through the blood vessels is called

_____.

7. The heart muscle contracts in two phases called the _____ _____.

8. The active phase of the cardiac cycle, during which the myocardium contracts, sending blood out of the heart, is called

_____.

9. The resting phase of the cardiac cycle, during which the myocardium relaxes, allowing the chambers to fill with blood, is called

_____.

10. A condition that results from pooling of blood in the veins just underneath the skin, causing them to become swollen and "knotty" in appearance, is called

_____.

THE NERVOUS SYSTEM

Key Learning Points

- Main parts of the nervous system
- Main functions of the nervous system
- Normal changes in the nervous system due to aging
- The words *central nervous system, peripheral nervous system, neuron, myelin, synapse, sensory nerves,* and *motor nerves*

Activity A *Place a "C" next to the structures that are a part of the central nervous system, and a "P" next to the structures that are a part of the peripheral nervous system.*

1. _____ Cerebellum
2. _____ Sensory nerves
3. _____ Diencephalon
4. _____ Motor nerves
5. _____ Brain stem
6. _____ Cerebrum
7. _____ Cranial nerves
8. _____ Spinal cord

Activity B *Fill in the blanks using the words given in parentheses.*

1. The nervous system helps to maintain the body's _____ (homeostasis/alignment) by controlling the other organ systems.

2. The nervous system allows us to interact with our _____ (neurons/environment) through the special senses of sight, hearing, smell, taste, and touch.

Activity C *Think About It! Briefly answer the following question in the space provided.*

Due to changes that occur with aging, older people tend to have slower reaction times. What does this put an older person at risk for?

_____

Activity D *Match the words, given in Column A, with their descriptions, given in Column B.*

Column A

_____ 1. Central nervous system

_____ 2. Peripheral nervous system

_____ 3. Neuron

_____ 4. Myelin

_____ 5. Synapse

_____ 6. Sensory nerves

_____ 7. Motor nerves

Column B

a. A cell that can send and receive information

b. Nerves that carry commands from the brain to the muscles and organs of the body

c. Consists of the brain and spinal cord

d. Nerves that carry information from the internal organs and the outside world to the spinal cord and up into the brain

e. Helps to speed the conduction of nerve impulses along the axon

f. Nerves outside of the brain and spinal cord;

g. Gap between the axon of one neuron and the dendrites of the next

THE SENSORY SYSTEM

Key Learning Points

- Main functions of the sensory system
- Senses of touch, position, and pain
- Senses of taste and smell
- Senses of sight
- Senses of sound
- Normal changes in the sensory system due to aging
- The words *sensory receptors, cerumen, presbyopia,* and *presbycusis*

Activity A *Fill in the blanks using the words given in parentheses.*

(general sense, sensory receptors, stimulus)

1. _____ are cells or groups of cells associated with a sensory nerve.

2. The sensory receptors pick up information, called a _____, and translate it into a nerve impulse.

3. The sensory receptors that are responsible for _____ are found throughout the body.

Activity B *Match the words, given in Column A, with their descriptions, given in Column B.*

Column A

_____ 1. Touch

_____ 2. Deep touch

_____ 3. Position

_____ 4. Pain

_____ 5. Taste and smell

Column B

a. Sensory receptors are found in the muscles, tendons, and joints.

b. Receptors are stimulated when something comes in contact with the surface of the body and presses on them, causing them to change shape.

c. Sensory receptors change a chemical signal into an electric one.

d. Some sensory receptors allow us to sense pressure.

e. Free nerve endings (dendrites) in the skin and the tissues of our internal organs

Activity C *Use the clues to complete the crossword puzzle.*

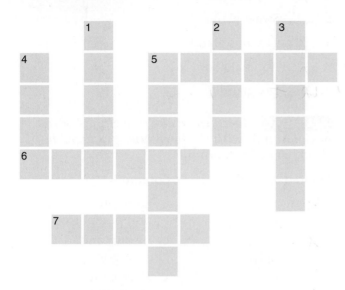

ACROSS

5. The clear, front portion of the eye that allows the light to pass through to the inside of the eye
6. The tough outer layer of the eye
7. Nerve that carries image from the retina to the brain

DOWN

1. An opening in the center of the iris
2. It controls the amount of light that enters the eye
3. It contains sensory receptors that turn light into nerve impulses
4. A flexible, transparent, curved structure in the eye that adjusts to focus light rays
5. The middle layer of the eye that contains the blood vessels

Activity D *Some of the steps that allow us to hear sounds are listed below. Write down the correct order of the steps in the boxes provided below.*

1. The tympanic membrane vibrations are passed to the first bone of the inner ear.

2. The malleus sends vibrations to the incus and then to the stapes.

3. Sounds travel in the form of sound waves, which are captured by the pinna and sent down the external auditory canal.

4. The stapes rests against the oval window, a membrane at the opening of the cochlea.

5. As the sound waves travel down the external auditory canal, they come in contact with the tympanic membrane, causing it to vibrate.

6. When the stapes vibrates, it causes the oval window to vibrate, sending the vibrations through the fluid inside the cochlea.

7. The moving fluid stimulates the receptors inside the cochlea, which then sends nerve impulses via the cochlear nerve to the brain.

8. The brain interprets these nerve impulses as sound.

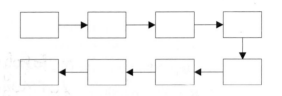

Activity E *Match the words/conditions, given in Column A, with their descriptions, given in Column B.*

Column A	Column B
_____ 1. Sensory receptors	a. Decrease in chemoreceptors on the tongue and roof of the nasal cavity
_____ 2. Cerumen	b. Age-related loss of the eye's ability to focus on objects that are close
_____ 3. Presbyopia	
_____ 4. Presbycusis	c. Specialized cells or groups of cells associated with a sensory nerve
_____ 5. Loss of sensory receptors in the skin	d. A waxy substance that helps to protect the external auditory canal
_____ 6. Decrease in appetite	e. Age-related hearing loss
	f. Risk for accidental burns

THE ENDOCRINE SYSTEM

Key Learning Points

- Main function of the endocrine system
- Glands that make up the endocrine system
- Hormones produced by the different glands of the endocrine system
- Normal changes in the endocrine system related to aging
- The word *hormones*

Activity A *Fill in the blanks using the words given in parentheses.*

(homeostasis, decrease, metabolism, chemicals, hormones, blood)

1. The endocrine system controls many of the body's processes, such as growth and development, reproduction, and _metabolism_

2. The endocrine system produces _hormones_ that are released into the bloodstream.

3. The hormone travels in the _blood_ until it reaches the specific cells that it acts on.

4. Hormones with short-term effects help the body to maintain _homeostasis_.

5. Hormones are _chemicals_ that act on cells to produce a response.

6. Many of the physical changes that are part of aging are directly related to a _decrease_ in the amount of hormones released throughout the body.

Activity B *Place an "X" next to the glands that are part of the endocrine system.*

1. _X_ Pituitary gland
2. _X_ Pineal gland
3. ____ Salivary gland
4. _X_ Thyroid gland
5. ____ Sweat gland
6. _X_ Thymus gland
7. _X_ Adrenal gland
8. _X_ Sex gland

Activity C *Match the endocrine glands, given in Column A, with the hormones produced by them, given in Column B.*

Column A	Column B
_c_ 1. Thyroid gland	a. Epinephrine and norepinephrine
_a_ 2. The medulla of the adrenal gland	b. Insulin and glucagon
_d_ 3. The cortex of the adrenal gland	c. Thyroxine and calcitonin
_b_ 4. The pancreas	d. Glucocorticoids, mineralocorticoids, and androgens

THE DIGESTIVE SYSTEM

Key Learning Points

- Main parts of the digestive system
- Main functions of the digestive system
- Normal changes related to aging that occur in the digestive system
- The words *feces, peristalsis, digestion, enzymes, absorption,* and *constipation*

Activity A *The figure shows the human digestive system. Label the organs that form a part of the digestive system, using the words given in parentheses.*

(ascending colon, pharynx, mouth, small intestine, rectum, jejunum, salivary glands, esophagus, transverse colon, stomach, descending colon, pancreas, gallbladder, large intestine, liver, duodenum, sigmoid colon, ileum, anus, cecum)

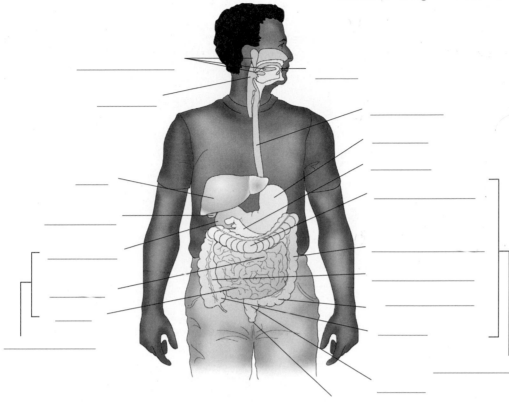

Activity B *Match the digestive organs, given in Column A, with their functions, given in Column B.*

Column A

_c__ 1. Teeth

_f__ 2. Esophagus

_e__ 3. Small intestine

_b__ 4. Liver

_a__ 5. Gallbladder

_d__ 6. Pancreas

Column B

a. Stores bile

b. Produces and secretes bile

c. Assists with chewing

d. Produces substances that aid in digestion, as well as insulin and glucagon

e. The mucus secreted by this organ, as well as the action of its muscle layer, helps to move food downward and into the stomach

f. Where most absorption of nutrients takes place

Activity C *Match the age-related changes, given in Column A, with their effects on the digestive system, given in Column B.*

Column A

_b__ 1. Missing or painful teeth

_c__ 2. Decrease in the production of saliva

_a__ 3. Slow movement of food through the digestive tract

Column B

a. Can put the older person at risk for constipation

b. Makes chewing difficult and increases the person's risk of choking

c. Makes swallowing difficult

Activity D ***Use the clues to complete the crossword puzzle.***

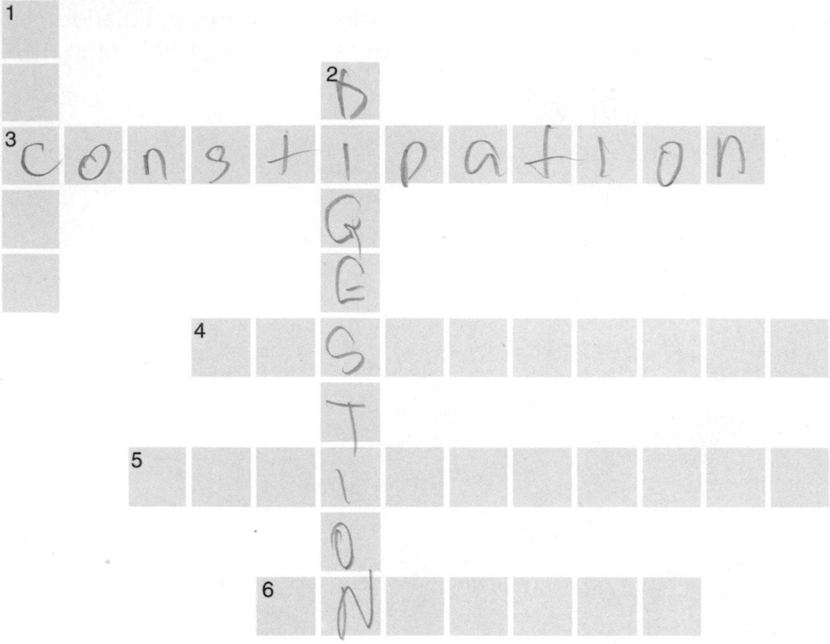
1
2
3
4
5
6
constipation
DIGESTION

ACROSS

3. A condition that occurs when the feces remain in the intestines for too long
4. Transfer of nutrients from the digestive tract into the bloodstream
5. Involuntary wavelike muscular movements
6. Substances that have the ability to break chemical bonds

DOWN

1. The semisolid waste product of digestion
2. The process of breaking food down into simple elements

THE URINARY SYSTEM

Key Learning Points

- Main parts of the urinary system
- Main functions of the urinary system
- Normal changes in the urinary system due to aging
- The words *filtrate* and *urine*

Activity A ***The figure shows the human urinary system. Label the figure using the words given in parentheses. Then, under the figure, briefly describe the function of each organ.***

(bladder, kidney, ureter, urethra)

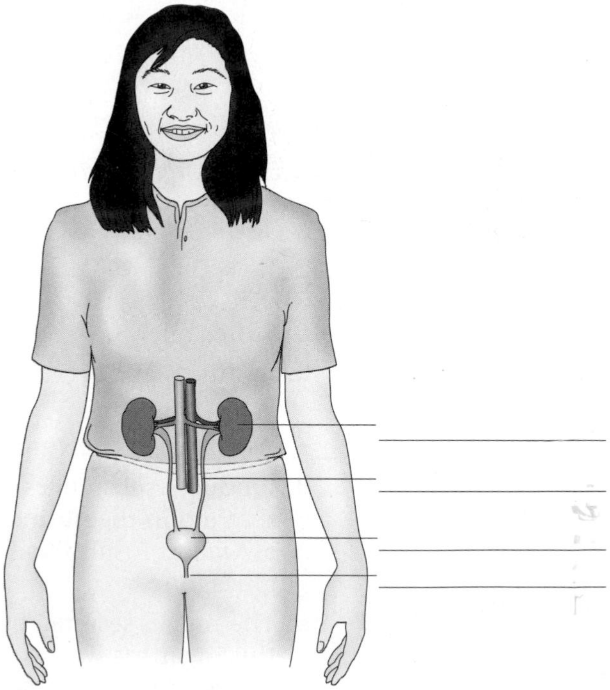

____

____

____

____

Activity B *Place an "X" next to statements that are true about the urinary system.*

1. _____ The urinary system consists of the kidneys, the ureters, the bladder, and the urethra.

2. _____ The main function of the urinary system is to remove waste products in the form of sweat.

3. _____ The urinary system removes waste products and excess fluid from the body in the form of urine.

4. _____ The urinary system helps to regulate the acidity of the blood.

5. _____ The normal functioning of the urinary system helps the body to maintain homeostasis.

Activity C *Match the age-related changes that occur in the urinary system, given in Column A, with their descriptions, given in Column B.*

Column A	Column B
_____ 1. Less efficient filtration	a. May result in episodes of overflow incontinence
_____ 2. Decreased muscle tone	b. Decrease in the kidneys' ability to filter waste products from the bloodstream
_____ 3. Enlargement of a man's prostate gland	c. Most common in older women who have had children or are obese; may contribute to stress incontinence

THE REPRODUCTIVE SYSTEM

Key Learning Points

- Main parts of the female reproductive system
- Main functions of the female reproductive system
- Main parts of the male reproductive system
- Main functions of the male reproductive system
- Normal changes occurring in the reproductive system due to aging

- The words *reproduction, sex cells, conception (fertilization), puberty, menopause, menstrual period, ovulation, lactation,* and *ejaculation*

Activity A *A figure of the female reproductive system is shown below. Label the figure using the words given in parentheses.*

(fallopian tube, cervix, uterus, ovary, vagina, fimbriae)

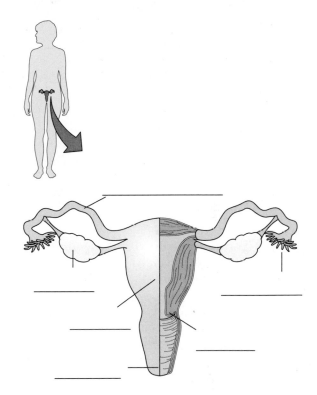

Activity B *Fill in the blanks using the words given in parentheses.*

(lactation, vagina, ovaries, uterus, fertilization)

1. The _____ contain all the eggs in a "holding pattern" until they are needed.

2. _____, if it occurs, occurs in the fallopian tubes.

3. The fertilized egg will attach to the lining of the _____ and continue to grow.

4. The _____ serves as the birth canal, through which a baby passes during birth.

5. When the breast tissue is stimulated by the hormone prolactin, _____ occurs.

Activity C *A figure of the male reproductive system is shown below. Label the figure using the words given in parentheses.*

(prostate gland, vas deferens, urinary bladder, testis, epididymis, penis, urethra, seminal vesicle)

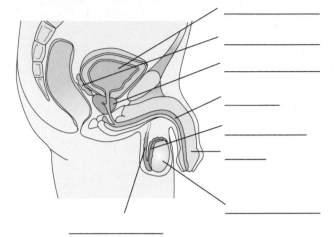

_____

Activity D *Match the organs of the male reproductive system, given in Column A, with their functions, given in Column B.*

Column A

_____ **1.** Testicles

_____ **2.** Epididymis

_____ **3.** Vas deferens

_____ **4.** Penis

Column B

a. Allows sperm cells to be deposited into the woman's reproductive tract

b. Sperm cells are mixed with the secretions from the seminal vesicles and the prostate gland.

c. The sperm cells mature and develop the whiplike "tail"

d. Secrete testosterone

Activity E *Place an "X" next to the correct statements.*

1. _____ Increased production of female sex hormones may also cause some women to develop facial hair.

2. _____ Menopause can cause "hot flashes," irritability, a loss of energy, and an inability to sleep.

3. _____ Some women experience vaginal dryness and irritation due to aging.

4. _____ Frequency and duration of erections in men decrease with age.

5. _____ Effects of aging on the respiratory system can result in decreased blood flow to the penis.

6. _____ The prostate gland in men tends to enlarge with age and make urination difficult.

Activity F *Fill in the blanks using the words given in parentheses.*

(puberty, conception, ovulation, ejaculation, menopause, sex cells, menstrual period, reproduction, lactation)

1. The process by which a living thing makes more living things like itself is called

_____.

2. _____ _____ are special cells contributed by each parent that contain half of the normal number of chromosomes.

3. _____ occurs when the male and female sex cells join, forming a cell that contains the complete number of chromosomes.

4. The period during which the secondary sex characteristics appear and the reproductive organs begin to function is called

_____.

5. _____ is the cessation of menstruation and fertility that women typically experience in their early 50s.

6. The monthly loss of blood through the vagina that occurs in the absence of pregnancy is called the _____ _____.

7. The release of a ripe, mature egg from the female ovaries each month is called

_____.

8. _____ is the process by which the glandular tissue of the female breast produces milk.

9. _____ is the forceful release of semen from the body.

Common Disorders

INTRODUCTION TO DISORDERS

Key Learning Points

- Acute and chronic disorders
- General categories used to describe the causes of disorders
- Factors that may put a person at risk for developing a certain disorder
- The words *disease, acute,* and *chronic*

Activity A *Fill in the blanks using the words given in parentheses.*

(acute, disease, chronic, homeostasis)

1. A disorder is something that affects the

   body's ability to maintain _____.

2. A/an _____ is a condition that occurs when the structure or function of an organ or organ system is abnormal.

3. A disorder with a rapid onset and a relatively short recovery time is called a/an

   _____ disorder.

4. A disorder that is ongoing and often needs to be controlled through continuous medication or treatment is called a/an

   _____ disorder.

Activity B *Match the type of disorder, given in Column A, with its cause, given in Column B.*

Column A

_____ **1.** Infectious

_____ **2.** Degenerative

_____ **3.** Nutritional

_____ **4.** Metabolic

_____ **5.** Immunologic

_____ **6.** Neoplastic

_____ **7.** Psychiatric

_____ **8.** Traumatic

Column B

a. The body is unable to metabolize or absorb certain nutrients, often the result of producing too much of one type of hormone, or not enough.

b. Germs invade the body.

c. The tissues of the body wear out or break down.

d. The body's ability to function is changed by an outside force.

e. The person's diet is out of balance.

f. The immune system does not work properly, the immune system may not be able to fight off infection, or the immune system starts to attack the body's own tissues.

g. A tumor invades otherwise healthy tissues and prevents the tissues from functioning properly.

h. The person is unable to maintain emotional balance.

Activity C *Mark each statement as either "true" (T) or "false" (F). Correct the false statements.*

1. T F Age does not influence how a person reacts to disease.

2. T F Some disorders are more common in men than in women, and vice versa.

3. T F The genes that we get from our parents may put us at risk for developing certain diseases.

4. T F A person's living conditions and health habits play a major role in the person's overall health status.

5. T F A person who has a chronic disease, such as diabetes or high blood pressure, is at reduced risk for developing another disease.

6. T F A person's emotional health does not affect his or her physical health.

INTEGUMENTARY DISORDERS

Key Learning Points

- Risk for infection due to integumentary system disorder
- Types of burns
- Types of lesions
- Nursing assistant's role in promoting comfort and skin healing in a person with a skin lesion
- The words *lesion* and *rash*

Activity A *Place an "X" beside those situations in which the person is at an increased risk for infection.*

1. _____ A person has suffered severe burns

2. _____ A person is in a health care facility for treatment of injuries that have immobilized her temporarily

3. _____ A person has a surgical wound

4. _____ A person has developed a pressure ulcer

5. _____ A person has intact skin and mucous membranes

Activity B *Match the type of burn, given in Column A, with its description, given in Column B.*

Column A

_____ **1.** First-degree burns

_____ **2.** Second-degree (partial-thickness) burns

_____ **3.** Third-degree (full-thickness) burns

Column B

a. Involve the epidermis and dermis, the subcutaneous layer, and often the underlying muscles and bones

b. Cause injury to the outermost layer of the skin, the epidermis

c. Penetrate into the dermis of the skin

Activity C *Use the clues to complete the crossword puzzle.*

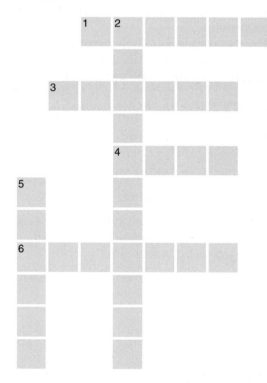

ACROSS

1. A general term used to describe any break in the skin
3. Small, flat, reddened lesions
4. A group of lesions
6. Small, pus-filled, blister-like lesions

DOWN

2. An abrasion or a scraping away of the surface of the skin
5. Small, raised, firm bumps

Activity D *List four actions a nursing assistant can take to help promote comfort and skin healing in a person with a skin lesion.*

1. _____
2. _____
3. _____
4. _____

MUSCULOSKELETAL DISORDERS

Key Learning Points

- Caring for a person with osteoporosis
- Common types of arthritis
- Caring for a person who has had hip joint replacement surgery
- Methods of repairing fractures
- Caring for a person who has a cast
- Situations that can lead to amputation
- The terms *osteoporosis, arthritis, fracture, traction, amputation,* and *phantom pain*

Activity A *Think About It! Briefly answer the following question in the space provided.*

Mrs. Bradford has osteoporosis. What is osteoporosis? List four special considerations that you will have when caring for Mrs. Bradford.

Osteoporosis: _____

When caring for a person who has osteoporosis:

1. _____
2. _____
3. _____
4. _____

Activity B *Fill in the blanks using the words given in parentheses.*

(rheumatoid, osteoarthritis, joint replacement, arthritis)

1. _____ is an inflammation of the joints, usually associated with pain and stiffness.
2. _____ usually affects weight-bearing joints, such as the knees, hips, and joints of the spine.
3. _____ arthritis is an autoimmune disorder that can cause severe joint deformities.
4. People who have very severe osteoarthritis may need _____ _____ surgery.

Activity C *Think About It! Briefly answer the following question in the space provided.*

Mr. Whitman recently had a hip replacement surgery. What special considerations do you need to keep in mind when caring for Mr. Whitman?

_____
_____
_____
_____

Activity D *Mark each statement as either "true" (T) or "false" (F). Correct the false statements.*

1. T F A fracture is usually caused by trauma.
2. T F Young people are especially at risk for fractures.
3. T F A person who has broken a bone is said to have a rupture.
4. T F Traction is a treatment for fracture in which the ends of the broken bone are placed in the proper alignment and then weight is applied to exert a constant pull and keep the bone in alignment.
5. T F A cast is applied to a fracture that is not complicated and can be corrected by aligning the broken ends.

6. T F A complicated fracture may be corrected by surgery, using metal plates, screws, rods, pins, or wires to hold the broken ends of the bone in alignment.

7. T F A person with a cast should keep it clean and moist.

8. T F Observations of cyanosis, foul odor, swelling, or increased drainage on the cast should be reported immediately.

9. T F A person with a cast should be advised against inserting objects between the cast and the skin.

10. T F The part of the body that is in a cast should be elevated on a pillow for several days.

Activity E *Place an "X" next to the statements that are true.*

1. _____ An amputation may be necessary as a result of trauma or disease.

2. _____ Amputation may become necessary because of complications related to diabetes.

3. _____ The feeling that a body part is still present, after it has been surgically removed, is called phantom pain.

4. _____ Sensations such an itching or aching after an amputation are caused by the healing of the bones that were cut in the process.

RESPIRATORY DISORDERS

Key Learning Points

- Respiratory tract infections
- Collecting a sputum specimen
- Types of chronic obstructive pulmonary disease (COPD)
- General care measures that a nursing assistant may use to assist a person with a respiratory disorder

Activity A *Select the single best answer for each of the following questions.*

1. Mrs. Wells has pneumonia. What might be a nursing assistant's responsibility when caring for Mrs. Wells?

a. To order oxygen therapy to help Mrs. Wells to breathe

b. To gather knowledge about which microbe is causing the pneumonia

c. To give Mrs. Wells her antibiotics

d. To collect a sputum specimen for analysis

2. Which of the following conditions usually causes a productive cough?

a. Bronchitis

b. Asthma

c. Pneumonia

d. Emphysema

3. Why is it important for staff and residents of long-term care facilities to receive an annual "flu shot"?

a. Because influenza virus can cause serious complications in older people

b. Because infection with the influenza virus can lead to a serious liver disorder

c. Because the influenza virus can lead to an extremely severe form of asthma

d. Because infection with the influenza virus causes the fragile walls of the alveoli to break

4. Which of the following are signs and symptoms of influenza?

a. Fever, pain when breathing, cyanosis, and a productive cough

b. Sore throat, dry cough, stuffy nose, headache, body aches, weakness, and fever

c. Vomiting, diarrhea, and loss of appetite

d. Wheezing and difficulty breathing

5. Why does a person find an asthma attack very frightening?
   a. Because the airways can narrow to the point that breathing becomes almost impossible
   b. Because the person may have a seizure
   c. Because the treatment for asthma is very painful
   d. Because the person must use supplemental oxygen to carry out even the simplest activities of daily living

6. Which of the following can trigger an asthma attack?
   a. Stress
   b. Exercise
   c. Cold weather
   d. All of the above

7. Which lung disorders are described by the term *chronic obstructive pulmonary disease* (COPD)?
   a. Pneumothorax and hemothorax
   b. Chronic bronchitis and pneumonia
   c. Emphysema and chronic bronchitis
   d. Bronchitis and asthma

Activity B *Place an "X" next to the correct guidelines to be considered when collecting a sputum specimen.*

1. _____ The person should rinse the mouth with water before coughing up the specimen.

2. _____ Sputum for the specimen should be coughed up from deep down in the respiratory tract.

3. _____ The person should spit into some tissue and the sputum should then be transferred from the tissue into a specimen container.

4. _____ The person should rinse the mouth with mouthwash before coughing up the specimen.

Activity C *Fill in the blanks using the words given in parentheses.*

(barrel, emphysema, chronic bronchitis, tightness)

1. _____ is a form of COPD that results from damage to the alveoli.

2. The chest of a person with emphysema may be enlarged and rounded, also called _____ chest.

3. A person with _____ _____ has ongoing irritation of the bronchi, leading to the production of thick mucus, which blocks the flow of air through the airways.

4. A person with chronic bronchitis could complain of _____ in the chest.

Activity D *List three things that you can do to help a person with respiratory problems feel more comfortable.*

1. _____
2. _____
3. _____

Activity E *Solve the crossword puzzle using the clues given below.*

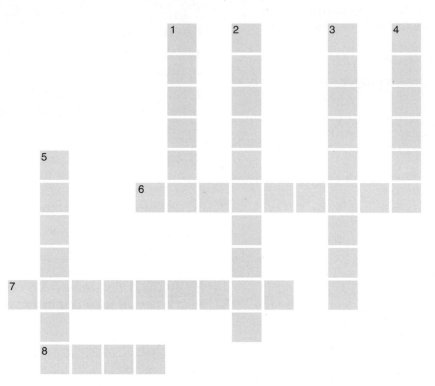

ACROSS

6. A disorder caused by long-term exposure of the alveoli to toxins, such as tobacco smoke; one of two forms of chronic obstructive pulmonary disease
7. An inflammation of the lung tissue, caused by infection with a virus or bacterium
8. Abbreviation of the general term used to describe two related lung disorders, emphysema and chronic bronchitis

DOWN

1. Mucus and other respiratory secretions that are coughed up from the lungs, bronchi, and trachea
2. Inflammation of the bronchi
3. An acute respiratory infection caused by the influenza virus
4. A condition that narrows the bronchi and bronchioles of the lungs, making breathing difficult
5. A type of bronchitis caused by long-term irritation of the bronchi and bronchioles, such as that caused by inhaling tobacco smoke; one of two forms of chronic obstructive pulmonary disease

CARDIOVASCULAR DISORDERS

Key Learning Points

- Disorders that affect the blood vessels
- Risk factors for developing heart disease
- Coronary artery disease
- Signs and symptoms of a myocardial infarction
- Use of pacemaker
- The words *atherosclerosis, plaque, embolus, arteriosclerosis, angina pectoris, myocardial infarction,* and *heart failure*

Activity A *Select the single best answer for each of the following questions.*

1. Plaque can build up on the inside of the wall of an artery, causing a condition called:
   a. Pulmonary embolus
   b. Arteriosclerosis
   c. Venous thrombosis
   d. Atherosclerosis

2. A person with venous thrombosis is at a higher risk of developing:

   a. Plaque

   b. An embolus

   c. Arteriosclerosis

   d. Varicose veins

Note: Disorders of the blood vessels include atherosclerosis and venous thrombosis. Both atherosclerosis and venous thrombosis put the person at risk for developing an embolus, a potentially fatal condition.

Activity B *Listed below are some of the risk factors for developing heart disease. Place a "Y" next to those factors that we CAN control, and place an "N" next to those factors we CANNOT control.*

1. _____ Smoking

2. _____ Gender

3. _____ Physical inactivity

4. _____ Obesity

5. _____ Heredity

6. _____ Diet high in fat

7. _____ Body build

8. _____ Poorly controlled hypertension

9. _____ Age

10. _____ Poorly controlled diabetes

Activity C *Place an "X" next to the correct statements.*

1. _____ Coronary artery disease occurs when the coronary arteries expand.

2. _____ People with angina pectoris may keep nitroglycerin pills on hand to relieve the pain when it occurs.

3. _____ A myocardial infarction occurs due to lack of blood and oxygen supply to the heart.

4. _____ A person who is experiencing angina may feel as though he is suffocating, and he may become very anxious.

5. _____ Anginal pain is only felt in the center of the chest.

Activity D *List five signs that may indicate that a person is having a myocardial infarction.*

1. _____

2. _____

3. _____

4. _____

5. _____

Activity E *Complete the statements below.*

1. What happens when the pathway that the heart uses to send the electrical impulse is blocked?

   _____

2. What happens when the heart rate of a person with a pacemaker drops below a programmed rate?

   _____

3. What happens when the pacemaker sends electrical impulses to the heart?

   _____

Activity F *Fill in the blanks with appropriate words from the list in brackets below.*

[embolus, angina pectoris, arteriosclerosis, plaque, myocardial infarction, atherosclerosis, heart failure]

1. A condition in which the arteries are blocked by plaque on the inside of the vessel wall is

   called _____.

2. Fatty deposits that build up on the inside of

   the artery wall are called _____.

3. A/an _____ is a blood clot in a vessel that breaks off and moves from one place to another.

4. A condition caused by hardening of the

   arteries is called _____.

5. The classic chest pain felt as a result of the heart muscle being deprived of oxygen is

   called _____ _____.

6. A/an _____ _____ occurs when one or more of the coronary arteries become completely blocked, preventing blood from reaching the parts of the heart that are fed by the affected arteries.

7. _____ _____ is a condition that occurs when the heart is unable to pump enough blood to meet the body's needs.

NERVOUS SYSTEM DISORDERS

Key Learning Points

- Difference between a transient ischemic attack (TIA) and a stroke
- Signs and symptoms of a stroke ("brain attack")
- Risk factors for having a stroke
- Effects of a stroke
- Effects of Parkinson's disease
- Effects of multiple sclerosis (MS) and amyotrophic lateral sclerosis (ALS, Lou Gehrig's disease)
- Effects of spinal cord injuries and head injuries
- The words *transient ischemic attack (TIA), stroke, hemiplegia, aphasia, Parkinson's disease, multiple sclerosis (MS), quadriplegia,* and *paraplegia*

Activity A *Place "TIA" next to statements that describe a transient ischemic attack and "S" next to statements that describe a stroke.*

1. _____ This condition occurs when blood flow to the brain is temporarily blocked.

2. _____ This condition causes the blood flow to the brain tissue to be blocked long enough for the brain tissue to die or become damaged.

3. _____ This condition can be caused by low blood pressure, certain medications, cigarette smoking, or standing up suddenly after lying down.

4. _____ The person usually recovers from this condition completely within 24 hours.

5. _____ The effects of this condition may be permanent.

Activity B *Place an "X" next to observations that may indicate a person has had a stroke.*

1. _____ Sudden confusion or disorientation

2. _____ Normal speech

3. _____ Drooling

4. _____ Drooping of the eyelids or corner of the mouth

5. _____ No change in blood pressure

6. _____ Tingling or numbness of an arm or leg or the side of the face

Activity C *List three risk factors that increase a person's chances of having a stroke.*

1. _____

2. _____

3. _____

Activity D *Fill in the blanks using the words given in parentheses.*

(pressure ulcers, aphasia, expressive aphasia, hemiplegia, receptive aphasia, brain, tissue)

1. The effects of a stroke depend on the area of the _____ that is affected and the amount of _____ that is damaged.

2. _____, or paralysis on one side of the body, is a common disability resulting from a stroke.

3. _____ is a general term for a group of disorders that affect a person's ability to communicate with others following a stroke.

4. A person with severe hemiplegia will need frequent repositioning to prevent

    _____ _____ from forming.

5. A person with _____ _____ has trouble forming words.

6. A person with _____ _____ may say "no" when he means "yes."

Activity E *Think About It! Briefly answer the following questions in the space provided.*

Mrs. Ingram has Parkinson's disease.

1. What is Parkinson's disease?

_____

_____

_____

2. List six signs and symptoms of Parkinson's disease that you would expect to see in Mrs. Ingram.

a. _____

b. _____

c. _____

d. _____

e. _____

f. _____

Activity F *Select the single best answer for each of the following questions.*

1. Amyotrophic lateral sclerosis is also known as:
   a. Parkinson's disease
   b. Lou Gehrig's disease
   c. MS
   d. Biplegia

2. Multiple sclerosis is thought to be caused by a/an:
   a. Viral infection
   b. Head injury
   c. TIA
   d. Autoimmune disorder

Activity G *Fill in the blanks using the words given in parentheses.*

(head, paraplegia, brain, spinal cord, quadriplegia, tumors)

1. _____ damage can result from falls, accidents, gunshot wounds, and events that cause a person to stop breathing for a period of time.

2. A person with paralysis from the neck down is said to be affected with _____.

3. People with _____ injuries may develop seizures, memory problems, or behavioral problems.

4. A person affected with _____ is paralyzed from the waist down.

5. An injury to the _____ _____ in the neck area can result in quadriplegia.

6. Injuries to the spinal cord may be due to trauma, birth defects, or _____ of the spine.

SENSORY DISORDERS

Key Learning Points

- Cataracts and glaucoma
- Caring for a person who is blind
- Special measures to help a person who is deaf
- The words *cataract, glaucoma,* and *Braille*

Activity A *Mark each statement as either "true" (T) or "false" (F). Correct the false statements.*

1. T F A person's vision becomes more and more cloudy as a cataract worsens.

2. T F Glaucoma occurs when the aqueous humor in the anterior chamber of the eye is not reabsorbed into the bloodstream.

3. T F As more and more aqueous humor is formed, pressure builds up in the eye, squeezing the nerves and the blood vessels in the retina.

4. T F If cataracts are not treated, pressure can destroy the nerves, and vision is lost.

5. T F Many people with cataracts have surgery to remove the cloudy lens and replace it with an artificial one.

Activity B *Think About It! Briefly answer the following question in the space provided.*

Miss Scott, a resident at the nursing home where you work, is blind. List six guidelines that a nursing assistant should keep in mind when helping Miss Scott.

1. _____

2. _____

3. _____

4. _____

5. _____

6. _____

Activity C *Give an example of what may be available to assist a deaf person with the following activities.*

1. Speaking

   _____

2. Communicating by telephone

   _____

3. Watching television

   _____

4. Using ringing devices like a doorbell, alarm clock, telephone, and smoke alarm

   _____

Activity D *Unscramble the words using the clues given.*

1. The gradual yellowing and hardening of the lens of the eye.

   ACATCART   _____

2. A disorder of the eye that occurs when the pressure within the eye is increased to dangerous levels.

   AMUCGAOL   _____

3. A system that uses letters made from combinations of raised dots that allow a blind person to read.

   LIARBEL   _____

ENDOCRINE DISORDERS

Key Learning Points

- Difference between hyperthyroidism and hypothyroidism
- Difference between type 1 diabetes mellitus and type 2 diabetes mellitus
- Importance of monitoring blood glucose levels in people with type 1 diabetes mellitus
- Signs and symptoms that indicate that a person's blood glucose is not normal
- Importance of eating regular, nutritious meals and snacks for people with diabetes mellitus
- The words *diabetes mellitus, hypoglycemia,* and *hyperglycemia*

Activity A *Place an "X" next to the phrases that describe signs and symptoms of hyperthyroidism, and a "√" next to the phrases that describe signs and symptoms of hypothyroidism.*

1. _____ Weight loss

2. _____ Weight gain

3. _____ Intolerance to cold

4. _____ Sweating

5. _____ Irregular heartbeat

Activity B *Fill in the blanks using the words given in parentheses.*

(brain, diabetic coma, hyperglycemia, diabetes mellitus, hypoglycemia, pancreas, glucose, insulin)

1. _____ _____ is an endocrine disorder that results when the pancreas is unable to produce enough insulin.

2. Type 1 diabetes occurs when the cells in the

   _____ that produce insulin are destroyed.

3. A person with type 1 diabetes must receive

   daily injections of _____.

4. A drop in blood glucose levels is

   called _____.

5. A state of having too much glucose in the bloodstream is called _____.

6. People who are taking insulin need to have their blood _____ levels monitored closely.

7. Too little insulin results in hyperglycemia, which can lead to _____ _____ and death.

8. Too much insulin causes hypoglycemia, which robs the _____ of the glucose that it needs to function.

Activity C *List symptoms that show that a person's blood glucose level is not normal.*

_____

_____

_____

_____

Activity D *Think About It! Briefly answer the following question in the space provided.*

You are caring for Tanya, who has type 1 diabetes. Tanya receives two insulin injections each day. Why is it important to serve meals and snacks to Tanya at the scheduled time?

_____

_____

_____

DIGESTIVE DISORDERS

Key Learning Points

- Symptoms of a person with an ulcer
- Symptoms of a person with gallbladder disease
- Symptoms of a person with cancer involving the digestive system
- Types and effects of hepatitis
- The word *hepatitis*

Activity A *Listed below are symptoms that indicate cancer, ulcer, and gallbladder disorders. Place a "C," "U," or "G," respectively, in front of the statements that indicate the symptoms of that particular disorder.*

1. _____ The person may experience stomach pain, especially within 3 hours of eating.

2. _____ The person may experience episodes of severe pain in the upper abdominal region, which may spread to the back and shoulder on the person's right side.

3. _____ The person may experience loss of appetite, indigestion, pain, vomiting, constipation, changes in bowel movements, or blood in the stool.

4. _____ The person may feel uncomfortably full or nauseous after eating.

5. _____ The person may have indigestion, especially after eating foods that are high in fat.

Activity B *Fill in the blanks using the words given in parentheses.*

(liver, toxic, hepatitis, transplant)

1. _____ is an inflammation of the liver commonly caused by a viral infection.

2. Chemicals, drugs, and alcohol can also affect the _____.

3. If liver failure is severe, the person will die unless he or she receives a liver

_____.

4. The liver removes _____ substances from the bloodstream.

URINARY DISORDERS

Key Learning Points

- Common disorders of the urinary system
- Signs and symptoms that indicate urinary system disorder
- Caring for a person with kidney (renal) failure
- The word *dialysis*

Activity A *Match the disorders of the urinary system, given in Column A, with their description, given in Column B.*

Column A

_____ **1.** Infections

_____ **2.** Kidney stones

_____ **3.** Renal failure

Column B

a. The kidneys are unable to filter blood

b. They can affect any part of the urinary system

c. Clumps of minerals that form in the kidneys and bladder

Activity B *List the signs and symptoms, related to the factors listed, that could indicate a urinary system disorder.*

1. Urine: _____

2. Urination habits: _____

3. Physical discomfort: _____

Activity C *The following statements are about a person with kidney failure. Mark each statement as either "true" (T) or "false" (F). Correct the false statements.*

1. T F Dialysis is a procedure that is done to remove waste products and fluids from the body when a person's kidneys fail and can no longer perform this task.

2. T F It is important to measure and record urine output when a person is affected by kidney failure.

3. T F Vital signs are not as important as measuring urine output.

4. T F It is important to provide frequent skin care to a person with kidney failure.

5. T F The person's food and fluid intake should be monitored and recorded.

REPRODUCTIVE SYSTEM DISORDERS

Key Learning Points

■ Sexually transmitted diseases (STDs) that may affect the male or female reproductive systems

■ Cancers that may affect the male or female reproductive systems

■ The words *sexually transmitted disease (STD)* and *postmenopausal bleeding*

Activity A *Match the sexually transmitted diseases, given in Column A, with their descriptions, given in Column B.*

Column A

_____ **1.** Genital herpes

_____ **2.** Gonorrhea

_____ **3.** Chlamydia

_____ **4.** Human papillo-mavirus (HPV)

_____ **5.** Syphilis

Column B

a. May cause no signs or symptoms, but can cause infertility in both men and women

b. A painless lesion on the genitals that can lead to cardiovascular and neurological problems in later stages

c. Painful blisters around the vaginal opening and perineum

d. Greenish discharge from the urethra in men

e. May cause cervical cancer in women

Activity B *Place an "M" next to cancers that affect the male reproductive system and "F" next to cancers that affect the female reproductive system.*

1. _____ Ovarian cancer

2. _____ Prostate cancer

3. _____ Penile cancer

4. _____ Endometrial cancer

5. _____ Cervical cancer

6. _____ Testicular cancer

Activity C *Select the best single answer to each of the following questions.*

1. Which of the following sexually transmitted diseases can involve the whole body?

a. AIDS

b. Gonorrhea

c. Genital herpes

d. Chlamydia

2. Postmenopausal bleeding may be the first sign of which condition?

  a. Pregnancy

  b. Cervical cancer

  c. Endometrial cancer

  d. Ovarian cancer

MENTAL HEALTH DISORDERS

Key Learning Points

- Common mental health disorders
- Emotional challenges and their effect on an elderly person's mental health
- The words *coping mechanisms, defense mechanisms, depression, suicide, anxiety, delusions,* and *hallucinations*

Activity A *Fill in the blanks using the words given in parentheses.*

(defense, mental, coping, suicide, anxiety, hallucinations, depression, delusions, schizophrenia, bipolar)

1. _____ health disorders affect a person's mind, causing the person to act in unusual ways, experience emotional difficulties, or both.

2. Conscious and deliberate ways of dealing with stress, such as exercising, praying, or enjoying a hobby, are called _____ mechanisms.

3. _____ mechanisms are unconscious ways of dealing with stress.

4. _____ is an alteration in a person's mood that causes him or her to lose pleasure or interest in all usually pleasurable activities, such as eating, working, or socializing.

5. _____ is the act of taking one's own life intentionally and voluntarily.

6. _____ is the feeling of uneasiness, dread, apprehension, or worry.

7. False ideas or beliefs (especially about oneself) are called _____.

8. _____ are episodes when a person sees, feels, hears, or tastes something that does not really exist.

9. _____ disorders cause a person to have mood swings.

10. A person with _____ has trouble determining what is real and what is imaginary.

Activity B *Select the best single answer for the following question.*

1. Mrs. Walker, a resident at your facility, is 72 years old. You think she may be depressed because several of her friends have died recently, and you have noticed a change in her behavior. For example, she used to like to go to the activity room, but now whenever you try and get her to come to an activity, she gives you an excuse for not going. Based on your suspicions, what should you do?

  a. Be supportive of Mrs. Walker and wait for her mood to improve. She is grieving for the loss of her friends.

  b. Assume that Mrs. Walker is just getting older, and her behavior is a normal part of getting older.

  c. Report your observations to the nurse. Mrs. Walker could be suffering needlessly.

  d. Try to cheer Mrs. Walker up by bringing her special treats.

Rehabilitation and Restorative Care

INTRODUCTION TO REHABILITATION AND RESTORATIVE CARE

Key Learning Points

- Goal of rehabilitation
- Members of the rehabilitation team
- OBRA requirements for rehabilitative services
- The words *disability, rehabilitation,* and *restorative care*

Activity A *Fill in the blanks using the words given in parentheses.*

(disabilities, restorative, abilities, rehabilitation)

1. Rehabilitation helps a person learn to

   manage his _____ .

2. The goal of _____ is to return the person to a level of functioning that allows him to live as independently as possible.

3. Rehabilitation is achieved through

   _____ care.

4. Rehabilitation focuses on the individual

   needs and _____ of the patient or resident.

Activity B *Rehabilitation is a team effort started as soon as possible after the person's medical condition stabilizes. List the members who could be a part of the rehabilitation team.*

_____

_____

_____

Activity C *State the OBRA requirements concerning rehabilitative services.*

_____

_____

Activity D *Match the words, given in Column A, with their descriptions, given in Column B.*

Column A	Column B
_____ 1. Disability	a. Measures taken by health care workers to help a person with a disability to regain health, strength, and function
_____ 2. Rehabilitation	b. Impaired physical or emotional function
_____ 3. Restorative care	c. The process of helping a person with a disability to return to his or her highest level of physical, emotional, or economic function

TYPES OF REHABILITATION

Key Learning Points

■ Types of rehabilitation
■ The words *supportive devices, assistive devices, prosthetic devices,* and *contractures*

Activity A *Place an "X" next to the statements that are true.*

1. What are the purposes of physical rehabilitation?

_____ **a.** Helping a person to be emotionally stable

_____ **b.** Teaching a person how to use supportive devices

_____ **c.** Preventing complications due to immobility

_____ **d.** Using exercise to help strengthen a person's muscles

2. What is emotional rehabilitation?

_____ **a.** Assisting a person to adjust to living with a disability

_____ **b.** Helping a person to overcome suicidal thoughts

_____ **c.** Helping a person with a disability to learn to use a new mode of transport

_____ **d.** Assisting a person to cope with the losses caused by a disability

3. How does vocational rehabilitation assist a person with a disability?

_____ **a.** It helps a person to relearn old skills.

_____ **b.** It helps a person to find a new job to match her abilities.

_____ **c.** It helps a person to learn new job-related skills.

_____ **d.** It helps a person to be financially independent.

Activity B *Mark each statement as either "true" (T) or "false" (F). Correct the false statements.*

1. **T F** Assistive devices are artificial replacements for legs, feet, arms, or other body parts.

2. **T F** Supportive devices help to stabilize a weak joint or limb.

3. **T F** A person is said to have contractures when he has a permanent loss of motion in the joint.

4. **T F** Prosthetic devices are used by people who may have lost an arm or a leg.

5. **T F** Vocational rehabilitation is important to prevent contractures.

THE ROLE OF THE NURSING ASSISTANT

Key Learning Points

■ Responsibilities of the nursing assistant in providing restorative care
■ Reporting observations when providing restorative care

Activity A *Complete the following statements about the nursing assistant's responsibilities for providing restorative care, using the answer choices a–d.*

a. it is important for the person's self esteem to complete a task with minimal help.

b. to prevent complications of immobility.

c. to deal effectively with the person's anger or frustration.

d. to give the person an emotional boost and encourage him to keep working.

1. Assistance with repositioning is important

_____

2. It is important to celebrate even the smallest accomplishments _____

3. Assistance is offered only as needed

because_____

4. The nursing assistant must be empathetic

_____

Activity B *Place an "X" next to observations that should be reported to the nurse when providing restorative care.*

1. ____ There is a change in the person's abilities.

2. ____ The person repeatedly talks about suicide.

3. ____ A supportive device is broken or not working properly.

4. ____ The person has pain, swelling, or redness around supportive or prosthetic devices.

5. ____ There is no change in vital signs during or after the rehabilitation activity.

CHAPTER 10

Infection Control

CAUSES OF INFECTION

Key Learning Points

- Types of germs that can cause disease
- Conditions that promote the growth of germs
- The words *microbe* and *pathogen*

Activity A *Mark each statement as either "true" (T) or "false" (F). Correct the false statements.*

1. T (F) Pathogens or germs are harmless microbes.

2. (T) F Microbes are living things that cannot be seen with the naked eye.

3. (T) F Microbes can be classified as bacteria, viruses, fungi, or parasites.

4. T (F) Urinary tract infections are usually caused by a virus.

5. (T) F Ringworm is caused by fungi.

Activity B *Place an "X" next to the conditions that promote the growth of germs.*

1. _____ Dry environment
2. _____ Well-lighted environment
3. _X_ Warm environment
4. _X_ Moist environment
5. _____ Clean environment
6. _X_ Dark environment

DEFENSES AGAINST INFECTION

Key Learning Points

- Defense mechanisms used by the body to fight infection
- The word *antibodies*

Activity A *Fill in the blanks using the words given in parentheses.*

1. _Non Specific_ (Specific/Nonspecific) defense mechanisms help to protect us from all infections.

2. _Specific_ (Specific/Nonspecific) defense mechanisms help to protect us only from certain infections.

3. Our first lines of defense against infections include healthy skin and _antibiotics_ _____. (antibiotics/mucous membranes)

4. Clean, dry _skin_ (skin/membranes) without cuts or wounds prevents pathogens from entering the body.

5. Sticky _____ (mucus/skin) traps and destroys pathogens.

6. The _____ (increased/decreased) blood flow to an infected area causes the area to become red, hot, swollen, and painful.

7. _____ (Mucus/Fever) causes the pathogen's environment to become too hot and the pathogen dies.

8. Our bodies produce _____ (antibodies/antibiotics) following exposure to certain pathogens.

9. _____ (Antivirals/Antibiotics) are used to treat bacterial infections.

10. _____ (Antiviral/Antimicrobial) agents are used to treat fungal and parasitic infections.

11. _____ (Antibiotic/Antiviral) agents are used to treat viral infections.

WAYS INFECTIONS ARE TRANSMITTED

Key Learning Points

- Airborne route of transmission
- Direct route of transmission
- Oral–fecal route of transmission
- Bloodborne route of transmission
- Body fluids that are most likely to contain bloodborne pathogens
- The words *airborne pathogens, oral–fecal route, bloodborne pathogen,* and *body fluids*

Activity A *Match the methods of transmission of infection, given in column A, with their descriptions, given in column B.*

Column A	Column B
_____ **1.** Airborne	**a.** Pathogen can be spread when an uninfected person touches an infected person
_____ **2.** Direct	
_____ **3.** Oral-fecal	**b.** Pathogen lives in an infected person's digestive tract and leaves the body in feces
_____ **4.** Bloodborne	
	c. Pathogen can be transmitted through blood or body fluids
	d. Pathogen can be spread through the air when a person coughs or sneezes

Activity B *List the body fluids that are most likely to contain bloodborne pathogens.*

_____

_____

THE CHAIN OF INFECTION

Key Learning Points

- Conditions that must be met for an infection to be spread from one person to another
- Breaking the chain of infection

Activity A *There are six key elements in the chain of infection that are essential for an infection to spread. Complete the following diagram with the six key elements that must be present for an infection to spread. We have filled in one to get you started.*

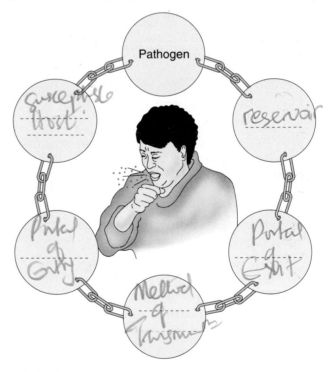

Activity B *The chain of infection can be broken by removing just one of the six elements that must be present for an infection to occur. Match each link in Column A with the action in Column B that will remove it, breaking the chain of infection.*

Column A

_____ 1. Reservoir

_____ 2. Portal of exit

_____ 3. Method of transmission

_____ 4. Portal of entry

_____ 5. Susceptible host

Column B

a. Covering an infected wound with a dressing

b. Washing your hands and making sure that linen, utensils, glassware, and other contaminated items are properly cleansed

c. Wearing gloves and keeping your skin healthy and intact

d. Receiving required immunizations and maintaining general good health

e. Taking the right antibiotic for a bacterial infection

METHODS OF INFECTION CONTROL

Key Learning Points

- Acquiring an infection within the health care system
- Four major methods of infection control
- Four techniques that make up the practice of medical asepsis
- Importance of handwashing in preventing the spread of infection
- Use of personal protective equipment (PPE) in infection control
- Use of isolation precautions to help prevent the spread of infection
- Use of airborne precautions, droplet precautions, contact precautions, and standard precautions
- Tuberculosis as a risk to health care workers
- Diseases caused by bloodborne pathogens that pose a special risk to health care workers and the effect of the viruses on the body
- Proper handwashing, gloving, masking, gowning, and double-bagging techniques

Activity A _Think About It! Briefly answer the following question in the space provided._

What factors make people more susceptible to getting infections in the health care setting?

_____

_____

_____

Activity B _Fill in the blanks using the words in parentheses._

(barrier methods, isolation precautions, surgical asepsis, medical asepsis)

1. The goal of _____ _____ is to remove pathogens from surfaces, equipment, and the hands of health care workers.

2. _____ _____ is used for surgical procedures, injections, inserting intravenous (IV) catheters, and inserting urinary catheters.

3. _____ _____ involve the use of personal protective equipment to prevent a pathogen from gaining access to a health care worker's body.

4. _____ _____ are guidelines followed to contain pathogens and limit others' exposure to them as much as possible.

Activity C _The following figure shows four techniques that make up the practice of medical asepsis. Identify the four techniques used in the figure and label them. Also write down their definitions._

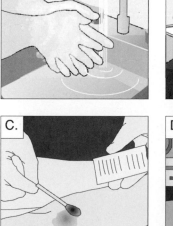
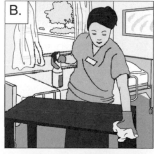
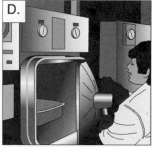

A. _____

B. _____

C. _____

D. _____

Activity D *Mark each statement as either "true" (T) or "false" (F). Correct the false statements.*

1. **T F** Handwashing does little to stop the spread of infection.

2. **T F** Transient flora can be easily transferred to the next patient or resident you care for, yourself, or one of your family members.

3. **T F** Most health care–associated infections (HAIs) are caused by transient flora.

4. **T F** Transient flora are difficult to remove.

5. **T F** You should wash your hands properly before entering a "clean" supply room.

6. **T F** Hands should be washed properly before obtaining clean linen from a linen cart or before handling a meal tray.

7. **T F** It is important to wash your hands before going on break and before leaving your shift.

8. **T F** It is not necessary to wash your hands after removing disposable gloves.

9. **T F** Always wash your hands after coughing, sneezing, blowing your nose, or touching your hair or applying make-up.

10. **T F** Wash your hands before entering a patient's or resident's room.

Activity E *Personal protective equipment (PPE) is worn to create a barrier between the health care worker and pathogens. List the items that are considered PPE and state when they should be worn.*

_____

_____

_____

_____

Activity F *Fill in the blanks using the words given in parentheses.*

(standard, bloodborne, pathogens, transmission-based)

1. Isolation precautions are guidelines that we follow to contain _____ and limit others' exposure to them as much as possible.

2. _____ precautions are used when a person is known or thought to have an infection that is transmitted by air, droplets, or contact.

3. Diseases caused by _____ pathogens are potentially life-threatening.

4. _____ precautions must be used with every patient or resident. For these methods to be effective, they must be used consistently.

Activity G *Place an "A" next to situations in which you would take airborne precautions, a "D" next to droplet precautions, and a "C" next to contact precautions. Also state the precautions you would take in each situation.*

1. _____ You are caring for a person who is suffering from whooping cough.

_____

2. _____ You have to change the soiled linens of a person with a draining wound.

_____

3. _____ You are caring for a person infected with measles.

_____

4. _____ You are helping an incontinent person to change her clothes.

_____

Activity H *Mark each statement as either "true" (T) or "false" (F). Correct the false statements.*

1. T F Tuberculosis (TB) is a disease that affects a person's liver.

2. T F Tuberculosis (TB) is spread when a person coughs, sneezes, speaks, or sings.

3. T F People who have close, frequent contact with a person who has tuberculosis (TB) are least likely to get the disease.

4. T F Health care workers are not at risk for getting tuberculosis (TB) from patients or residents.

Activity I *Mark each statement as either "true" (T) or "false" (F). Correct the false statements.*

1. T F Hepatitis B, hepatitis C, and hepatitis D cause inflammation of the liver.

2. T F People with chronic hepatitis B infection may never have symptoms, but they can still pass the virus on to others.

3. T F The illness that results from infection with HBV tends to be more chronic and serious than that resulting from infection with HCV.

4. T F Many people with HCV will eventually require a liver transplant in order to save their lives.

5. T F Vaccination against HBV protects against HDV.

6. T F HBV invades the body's T cells and uses it to make copies of itself and increase its numbers.

7. T F In a person with HIV infections, the number of T cells in the body decreases, and the body is unable to fight off infections.

8. T F Your chances of becoming infected with HIV on the job is much higher than your chances of becoming infected with HBV or HCV.

Bloodborne diseases that pose the most risk to health care workers include hepatitis B, hepatitis C, hepatitis D, and HIV/AIDS. The viruses that cause these diseases are found in body fluids.

Activity J *Fill in the blanks using the words given in parentheses.*

1. Stand _____ _____ (away from/close to) the sink when washing hands.

2. While washing hands, lather at least one inch past your wrists, keeping your fingers pointed _____ (down/up) at all times.

3. Apply a small amount of _____ _____ (alcohol rub/hand lotion) to keep your skin supple and moist.

4. When removing gloves, first use one _____ (gloved/ungloved) hand to pull the glove off the other hand.

5. When removing gloves, slip two fingers from the _____ (gloved/ungloved) hand underneath the cuff of the remaining glove, at the wrist.

6. After the gown is rolled up, contaminated side _____ (inward/outward), dispose it in a facility-approved container.

7. The cuffs of the _____ (gown/gloves) should extend over the cuffs of the _____ (gown/gloves).

8. The top strings of the mask are securely tied behind the _____ (neck/head), and the bottom strings of the mask are securely tied behind the _____ (neck/head).

9. _____ (Sterile/Contaminated) items are secured in an isolation bag.

10. The double-bagging technique involves _____ (two/four) nursing assistants.

11. During the double-bagging procedure one nursing assistant holds a plastic bag cuffed over her hands, while another nursing assistant places the _____ (isolation/sterile) bag into it.

Activity K *Match the words, given in Column A, with their meanings, given in Column B.*

Column A

_____ 1. Health care–associated infection (HAI)

_____ 2. Medical asepsis

_____ 3. Transient flora

_____ 4. Contaminated

_____ 5. Personal protective equipment (PPE)

_____ 6. Tuberculosis (TB)

_____ 7. Standard precautions

Column B

a. Techniques that are used to physically remove or kill pathogens

b. Adjective used to describe an object that is soiled by pathogens

c. An airborne infection caused by a bacterium that usually infects the lungs

d. An infection acquired while in a hospital or other health care setting

e. Precautions, including the use of barrier methods, that a health care worker takes with each patient or resident to prevent contact with bloodborne pathogens

f. Microbes that are picked up by touching contaminated objects or people who have an infectious disease

g. Barriers such as gloves, gowns, masks, and protective eyewear that are worn to physically prevent microbes from reaching a health care provider's skin or mucous membranes

OSHA BLOODBORNE PATHOGENS STANDARD

Key Learning Points

- Standards set by the Occupational Safety and Health Administration (OSHA) to protect health care workers from exposure to bloodborne pathogens in the workplace
- Responsibility of the employer and the employee for maintaining the employee's safety in the workplace

Activity A *The Occupational Safety and Health Administration has set standards to protect health care workers from exposure to bloodborne pathogens in the workplace. List the responsibility of the employer and the employee in each area below.*

1. Training:

Employer's responsibility: _____

_____

Employee's responsibility: _____

_____

2. Hepatitis vaccination:

Employer's responsibility: _____

_____

Employee's responsibility: _____

_____

3. Personal protective equipment:

Employer's responsibility: _____

_____

Employee's responsibility: _____

_____

4. Environmental control methods:

    Employer's responsibility: _____

    _____

    Employee's responsibility: _____

    _____

5. Exposure control plan:

    Employer's responsibility: _____

    _____

    Employee's responsibility: _____

    _____

11

Workplace Safety

PROTECTING YOUR BODY

Key Learning Points

■ The ABC's of body mechanics
■ The proper use of body mechanics to promote safety and make the body more effective while working
■ The use of proper lifting technique to prevent back injuries
■ The terms *body mechanics, alignment, balance,* and *coordinated body movement*

Activity A *Select the single best answer for each of the following questions.*

1. Which of the following activities places physical stress on the nursing assistant's body?
   a. Assisting a person out of bed
   b. Recording a person's temperature
   c. Showing a person how to use the call light control
   d. Arriving late at work

2. Which of the following is one of the basic components of good body mechanics?
   a. Using the powerful muscles in your back to lift
   b. Using coordinated body movement
   c. Standing with your shoulders hunched
   d. Standing with your feet close together

3. When you are standing, which part of your body is the center of gravity?
   a. The torso
   b. The head
   c. The feet
   d. The thigh muscles

4. When lifting, remember to use the large muscles of your
   a. Back
   b. Hips and thighs
   c. Arms
   d. Chest

5. What work-related injury are nursing assistants most at risk for?
   a. Communicable infection
   b. Back injury
   c. Electrical shock
   d. Falls

Activity B *The figure shows a person who is holding her body in proper alignment. Draw an imaginary line that indicates the person is in good alignment.*

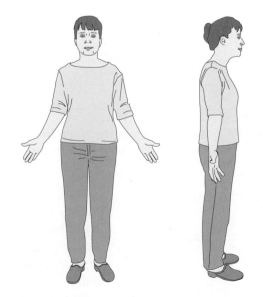

Activity C *Think About It! Briefly answer the following question in the space provided.*

You need to help Mr. Tompkins out of his wheelchair and into bed. List two ways you can stabilize your body and maximize your ability to remain balanced.

1. _____
   _____

2. _____
   _____

Activity D *The figure below shows good lifting technique. Write the correct order that the steps should be in, and describe each step.*

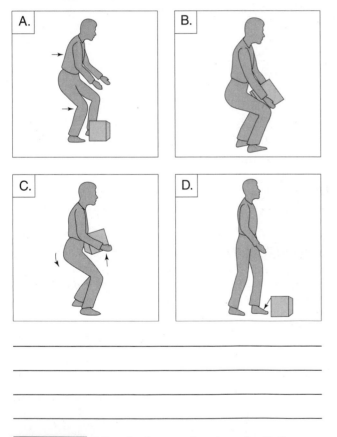

_____
_____
_____
_____
_____

Activity E *Match the words, given in Column A, with their meanings, given in Column B.*

Column A

1. _____ Alignment

2. _____ Body mechanics

Column B

a. Using the weight of the body to help with movement

b. Stability produced by even distribution of weight

3. _____ Coordinated body movement

4. _____ Balance

c. Good posture

d. The efficient and safe use of the body

FOLLOWING PROCEDURES

Key Learning Points

- Why nursing assistants follow procedures when providing patient or resident care
- The steps taken before every patient or resident care procedure
- The steps taken after every patient or resident care procedure
- The word *procedure*

Activity A *List the six pre-procedure or "getting ready" actions performed before every patient or resident care procedure.*

1. _____
2. _____
3. _____
4. _____
5. _____
6. _____

Activity B *List the six post-procedure actions or "finishing up" steps performed after every patient or resident care procedure.*

1. _____
2. _____
3. _____
4. _____
5. _____
6. _____

Activity C *Place an "X" next to the incorrect statements.*

1. _____ Only very complicated procedures require pre-procedure and post-procedure actions.

2. _____ Following procedures ensures only the patient's safety.

3. _____ Following recommended steps ensures both the patient's safety and yours, and makes procedures more efficient.

FIRE SAFETY

Key Learning Points

- The elements necessary for a fire to start and continue to burn
- Precautions taken in the health care setting to prevent fires
- The RACE fire response plan
- How to use a fire extinguisher

Activity A *The figure shows three elements that must be present for a fire to occur. Write the names of the three elements and list at least two sources of each below the figure.*

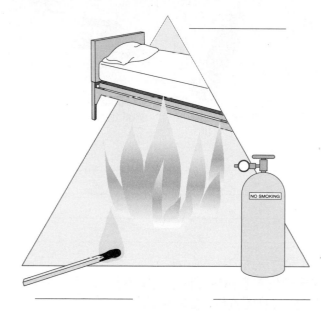

_____

_____

_____

_____

_____

Activity B *Match the type of extinguisher, given in Column A, with the type of fire that it is used to extinguish, given in Column B.*

Column A

_____ 1. Type A

_____ 2. Type B

_____ 3. Type C

Column B

a. Fire that is fueled by a petroleum product (e.g., gasoline, automotive oil), cooking oil, or grease

b. An electrical fire

c. Fire that is fueled by ordinary material such as wood, paper, cloth, leaves, and grass

Activity C *Write "YES" next to the type of fire that can be extinguished with water, and "NO" next to the type of fire that should not be extinguished with water.*

1. _____ Fire that is fueled by ordinary material such as wood, paper, cloth, leaves, and grass

2. _____ Fire that is fueled by a petroleum product (e.g., gasoline, automotive oil), cooking oil, or grease

3. _____ An electrical fire

Activity D *Think About It! Briefly answer the following question in the space provided.*

Miss Wray has an "oxygen in use" sign posted outside of her room. Why is it especially important to follow safety precautions designed to prevent fires when you are in Miss Wray's room?

_____

_____

_____

_____

Activity E *Look at the following pictures. Fill in the labels and the boxes for these events, according to the RACE fire response plan.*

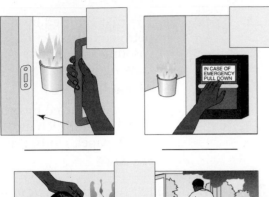

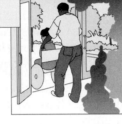

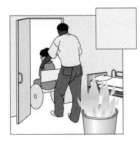

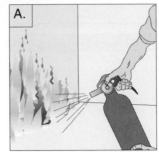
Spray the contents at the base of the fire.

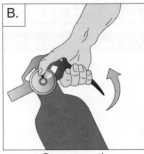
Squeeze the handle.

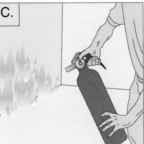
Aim the hose toward the base of the fire.

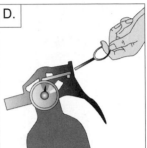
Pull the safety pin out.

Activity F *A fire has started in a wastebasket at the nurses' station. Look at the following pictures and write down the correct order of steps for using a fire extinguisher.*

1. _____

2. _____

3. _____

4. _____

PREVENTING CHEMICAL AND ELECTRICAL INJURIES

Key Learning Points

- Materials Safety Data Sheet (MSDS)
- Occupational Safety and Health Administration (OSHA) requirements
- How to handle a chemical properly and what to do in case of a chemical exposure
- Safety precautions that lower the risk of electrical shock and electrical fires

Activity A *What is a Materials Safety Data Sheet (MSDS)?*

_____

_____

_____

_____

Activity B *Knowing how to safely operate and maintain electrical equipment is necessary to prevent electrical shocks. Fill in the blanks using the words given in parenthesis.*

(frayed, grounded, power strip, loose, water)

1. Use _____ appliances, which have special three-prong plugs.

2. If more than two items must be plugged into an outlet, use a facility-approved

_____.

3. If you notice anything unsafe about an appliance that is being used, such as

_____ wires or _____ plugs, remove the appliance from use immediately.

4. Never operate electrical equipment around

_____.

Activity C *Mark each statement as either "true" (T) or "false" (F). Correct the false statements.*

1. T F OSHA requires employers to maintain a list of all chemicals used in their facility.

2. T F Employers need to maintain a list of only the toxic chemicals that are used in their facility.

3. T F The Materials Safety Data Sheet (MSDS) contains information about the chemicals that are used in the facility.

DISASTER PREPAREDNESS

Key Learning Points

- Disaster situations that may affect a health care facility
- The word *disaster*

Activity A *Think About It! Briefly answer the following question in the space provided.*

List five types of disasters that may affect a health care facility.

1. _____
2. _____
3. _____
4. _____
5. _____

Activity B *Define the word* disaster.

_____

_____

_____

CHAPTER 12

Patient and Resident Safety

ACCIDENTS IN THE HEALTH CARE SETTING

Key Learning Points

- Risk factors that may put people in a health care setting at a higher risk for accidents and injury
- Measures that a nursing assistant can take to prevent accidents in a health care facility
- How to assist a patient or resident who is falling
- The importance of reporting an accident and completing the necessary follow-up paperwork
- The word *incident (occurrence) report*

Activity A *Each of the people described in Column A is at risk for an accident. Match each person in Column A with his or her risk factor in Column B.*

Column A

_____ 1. Miss Janey has dementia.

_____ 2. Both of Mrs. Markus' knees are affected by arthritis, which makes it painful for her to walk.

_____ 3. Mr. Thompson uses glasses, which he often forgets to wear.

Column B

a. Poor mobility

b. Sensory impairment

c. Confusion and disorientation

Activity B *Select the single best answer for each of the following questions.*

1. Which of the following can cause confusion and disorientation?
   a. Dementia
   b. Head injury
   c. Medication reactions
   d. All of the above

2. You regularly assist Mrs. Martin to the facility garden in her wheelchair. One evening, she has an accident because her wheelchair brakes jam unexpectedly. Which of the following actions should you take?
   a. Avoid reporting the accident to the nurse because Mrs. Martin's injuries are minor and you can take care of them
   b. Report the accident immediately to the nurse and then fill out an incident (occurrence) report
   c. Report the accident to the doctor but not to the nurse
   d. Complete an incident (occurrence) report since the cause of the accident was equipment malfunction

3. Which of the following precautions would you take to avoid accidental burns to a person while bathing him or her?

a. Use cold water for the bath

b. Measure the temperature of the water with a bath thermometer before bathing the person

c. Allow the person to choose the water temperature

d. There is no need to take any precautions because the water heaters in the facility preset the water temperature for bathing.

Activity C *Think About It! Briefly answer the following question in the space provided.*

You are helping Mrs. Bowman to walk down the hall. Mrs. Bowman is recovering from pneumonia, and she is very weak and unsteady on her feet. All of a sudden, Mrs. Bowman starts to fall. Describe the steps you should take to help minimize your risk of injury, as well as Mrs. Bowman's.

1. _____
   _____

2. _____
   _____

3. _____
   _____

4. _____
   _____

Activity D *Think About It! Briefly answer the following question in the space provided.*

You are a home health aide caring for Mr. Warburton. Mr. Warburton is 87 years old and is in generally good health, but his family is concerned because he lives alone and they cannot check on him regularly. He has some problems with mobility. On your first visit to Mr. Warburton's house, you notice that Mr. Warburton likes to keep the shades drawn during the day, so the house is cool and dark. There are stacks of books and magazines everywhere, even on the floor. And when you open the refrigerator, you notice that most of the food in it has gone bad, but Mr. Warburton does not seem to be aware that the food is spoiled. You decide that you better report these observations to the nurse at the home health agency right away. What specific concerns do you have about Mr. Warburton's safety?

_____

_____

_____

Activity E *Mark each statement as either "true" (T) or "false" (F). Correct the false statements.*

1. T F Burns are the leading cause of accidental deaths among elderly people.

2. T F Before assisting a person with a reduced sense of touch with bathing, always check the temperature of the water by placing your hand in it.

3. T F An incident (occurrence) report is completed whenever an accident occurs in a health care facility.

Activity F *Sensory impairment can lead to serious accidents. Match the type of sensory impairment, given in Column A, with the accident it could cause, given in Column B.*

Column A	Column B
_____ 1. Reduced sense of touch	a. Mrs. Vincent overdosed on her medication
_____ 2. Poor vision	b. Mr. Watson suffocated due to a natural gas leak in his home
_____ 3. Reduced sense of smell and taste	c. Mrs. Vas, a resident with diabetes, suffered hot-water burns
_____ 4. Reduced sense of hearing and smell	d. Mr. Simon had food poisoning

Activity G *Think About It! Briefly answer the following question in the space provided.*

As a nursing assistant, you will take many measures to prevent your patients or residents from falling and injuring themselves. Briefly explain the reason for each of the following fall prevention guidelines.

1. Checking the patient's or resident's clothing and shoes.

   _____

   _____

2. Checking equipment used by the patient or resident, such as a wheelchair, cane, or walker.

   _____

   _____

3. Keeping the patient's or resident's bed as low as possible.

   _____

   _____

4. Removing clutter from walkways.

   _____

   _____

5. Immediately reporting to the nurse your observation that the person seems to have trouble with mobility.

   _____

   _____

6. Keeping a disoriented patient or resident who could be at a high risk of falling close to the nurses' station.

   _____

   _____

Activity H *Fill in the blank with the correct word.*

1. A preprinted document that is completed following an accident involving a patient or resident is called an _____ _____.

RESTRAINTS

Key Learning Points

- Why the use of restraints may sometimes be necessary in a health care setting
- The five different types of restraints
- Methods used to reduce the need for restraints
- Safety concerns of restraint use

- The proper application of a vest restraint, a wrist or ankle restraint, and a lap or waist (belt) restraint
- The words *physical restraint* and *chemical restraint*

Activity A *Select the single best answer for each of the following questions.*

1. Which one of the following statements describes the correct use of restraints?
   a. The restraint should be removed every 2 hours, for a total of 10 minutes.
   b. The restraint should be changed every day.
   c. If the patient or resident complains about the restraint, disregard the complaint because it is beyond the nursing assistant's scope of practice to remove a restraint.
   d. If the patient or resident complains about the restraint, disregard the complaint because the purpose of the restraint is to reduce the patient's or resident's risk for accidents.

2. Restraints are used for all of the following reasons EXCEPT:
   a. To provide postural support
   b. To protect the patient or a resident from harm
   c. To protect the staff from a combative patient or a resident
   d. For staff convenience

3. Which one of the following is your responsibility with regard to the use of restraints?
   a. To order a restraint for a patient or resident
   b. To provide care for the patient or a resident while he is in a restraint
   c. To administer a sedative to an agitated or combative patient or resident
   d. To remove a restraint at the patient's or resident's request

4. Each time you attend to a patient or a resident who is wearing a restraint, you should be alert to signs and symptoms related to the use of the restraint. Which of the following observations should you report to the nurse immediately?
   a. The restrained person is resting quietly.
   b. The restrained person's arm is cool to the touch and pale or blue.

c. The restrained person asks for a drink of water.

d. The restrained person has visitors.

Activity B *Write the name of the knot shown below and explain why this type of knot is used to secure a restraint.*

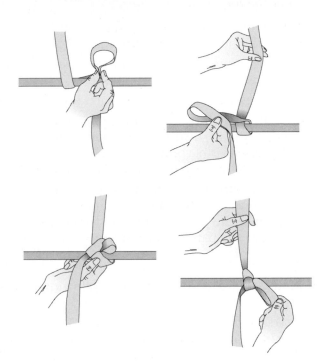

This knot is called a _____ knot. It is used to secure a restraint because

_____

_____

_____

Activity C *Write the name of the restraint shown in each figure below.*

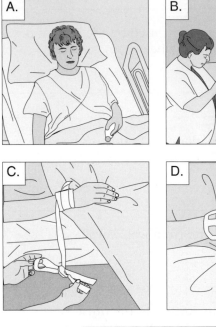
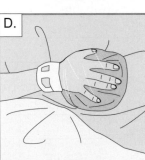
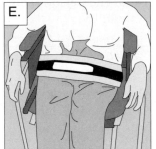
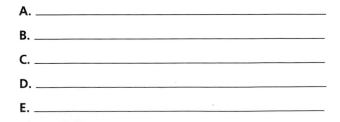

A. _____

B. _____

C. _____

D. _____

E. _____

Activity D *Think About It! Briefly answer the following questions in the space provided.*

What could happen if:

a. A vest restraint is put on backwards with the back of the vest on the person's chest and the flaps crossed across her back?

_____

b. A restraint is too tight?

_____

c. A person is left in a restraint for a long time?

_____

d. A person who is wearing a restraint is not taken to the bathroom regularly?

_____

Activity E *Think About It! Briefly answer the following question in the space provided.*

Restraints should only be used as a last resort. What are four things a nursing assistant can do to eliminate or reduce the need for restraints?

1. _____

2. _____

3. _____

4. _____

Activity F *The following are some of the steps used for applying a wrist restraint. Arrange the steps in the correct order by filling in the boxes below.*

a. Secure the restraint snugly, but not too tight. You should be able to slide two fingers under the restraint.

b. Report and record the procedure. Sign the chart and include your title and name.

c. Attach the straps to the bed frame. Always use the quick-release knot.

d. Reapply the restraint.

e. Get help from a nurse or another nursing assistant.

f. Meet the patient's needs for food, fluids and elimination. Give skin care and perform range-of-motion exercises.

g. If applying more than one restraint, repeat the steps.

h. Apply restraint following the manufacturer's instructions. Place the soft part of the restraint against the skin.

i. Check on the restrained person every 15 minutes and release the restraint every 2 hours.

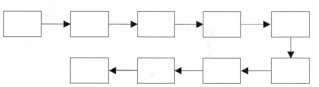

Activity G *Fill in the blanks using the words in parentheses.*

1. A _____ (physical/chemical) restraint is a device that is attached to or near a person's body to limit a person's freedom of movement or access to her body.

2. A _____ (physical/chemical) restraint is any medication that alters a person's mood or behavior, such as a sedative or tranquilizer.

CHAPTER 13

Basic First Aid and Emergency Care

RESPONDING TO AN EMERGENCY

Key Learning Points

- The nursing assistant's role in an emergency situation
- The words *disoriented, unresponsive,* and *basic life support*

Activity A *In the boxes provided below, write down the correct order of steps that you would take to help your neighbor in this emergency situation.*

Returning from work one day, you notice that your neighbor is lying in his yard next to a ladder and he's not moving! You rush over to assist him.

1. You activate the emergency medical services (EMS) system.

2. You gently touch your neighbor's shoulder and say, "Mr. Veracruz, are you OK?"

3. You recognize that an emergency exists.

4. You provide appropriate care until the EMS personnel arrive.

5. You decide to act.

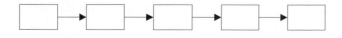

Activity B *Mark each statement as either "true" (T) or "false" (F). Correct the false statements.*

1. **T F** General training programs in basic emergency care are available and cover principles of first aid and basic life support (BLS).

2. **T F** Your familiarity with your patients or residents makes you less likely to notice signs and symptoms that could alert the health care team to the fact that there is a potential emergency situation.

3. **T F** When an emergency situation occurs, you should stay calm, organize your thoughts, and then act.

4. **T F** In case of an emergency, you should not speak to the patient or resident.

Activity C *Fill in the blanks using the words given in parentheses.*

(disoriented, unresponsive, basic life support)

1. A person who is unconscious and cannot be aroused, or who is conscious but does not react when spoken to or touched, is called

_____.

2. A person who is unable to answer basic questions about person, place, or time

is _____.

3. _____ includes basic emergency care techniques, such as rescue breathing and cardiopulmonary resuscitation (CPR).

BASIC LIFE SUPPORT (BLS) MEASURES

Key Learning Points

- The ABCs of emergency care
- The organizations that offer approved training in basic life support (BLS) measures
- The words *respiratory arrest* and *cardiac arrest*

Activity A *List the ABCs of emergency care.*

A. _____

B. _____

C. _____

Activity B *Select the single best answer for each of the following questions.*

1. What is the goal of basic life support (BLS)?

a. To prevent respiratory arrest

b. To prevent cardiac arrest

c. To keep a person who is in respiratory or cardiac arrest alive until help arrives

d. All of the above

2. Which of the following is an organization that offers approved training in basic life support (BLS) measures?

a. Blue Cross

b. Sisters of Mercy

c. American Heart Association

d. All of the above

3. The condition where breathing has stopped is called:

a. Cardiac arrest

b. Brain death

c. Shock

d. Respiratory arrest

Activity C

One day, you are driving down the highway when you see the car in front of you swerve suddenly. The car crashes through the guard rail and rolls down a small hill on the side of the road, landing upside down. You immediately pull over to assist the driver. By the time you get to the scene, another motorist has pulled the unconscious driver out of the car and away from the wreckage. You use your training to provide basic life support to the driver. Look at the following images depicting the steps of BLS and place them in the correct order.

A.
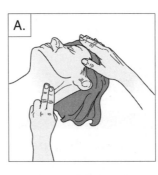

B.
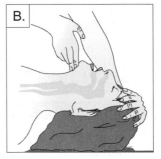

C.
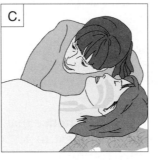

1. _____

2. _____

3. _____

EMERGENCY SITUATIONS

Key Learning Points

- How to assist a person who complains of feeling faint or who has fainted
- How to assist a person who is having a seizure
- How to assist a person who is bleeding uncontrollably (hemorrhaging)
- Some of the types and causes of shock, and how to assist a person who is in shock

- Situations that can put a person at risk for choking
- How to relieve an obstructed airway
- The words *syncope, epilepsy, hemorrhage, pulse points,* and *aspiration*

Activity A *Match the words, given in Column A, with their descriptions, given in Column B.*

Column A

_____ 1. Seizures

_____ 2. Fainting (syncope)

_____ 3. Hemorrhage

_____ 4. Shock

Column B

a. May be an early sign of a serious medical condition

b. Results when the organs and tissues of the body do not receive enough oxygen-rich blood

c. Occur when electrical brain activity is interrupted

d. Can be caused by trauma to a blood vessel or by certain illnesses, such as gastric ulcers

Activity B *Think About It! Briefly answer the following questions in the space provided.*

You are a home health care aide. One day, you are at a client's house and while you are cleaning the bathroom, the client decides to go downstairs to her basement. You hear a loud crash and a scream and when you go to investigate, you find that the client has fallen down the stairs and has a very deep wound on her leg, which is gushing blood.

1. What should you do first to help the client?

_____

_____

2. What should you do to control the blood loss until help arrives?

_____

_____

_____

_____

Activity C *Mark each statement as either "true" (T) or "false" (F). Correct the false statements.*

1. T F If you believe that a person is about to faint, loosen any restraints or tight clothing, and have the person remain in the supine or sitting position.

2. T F A person who is having a seizure may simply stop speaking and stare into space.

3. T F Seizures can cause a loss of consciousness and, because of the violent jerking of the muscles, the person who is having the seizure is at a risk for injuring herself.

4. T F Anaphylactic shock is caused by severe bacterial infections that involve the entire body.

5. T F People who are not conscious are not at risk for aspiration.

Activity D *Use the clues to complete the crossword puzzle.*

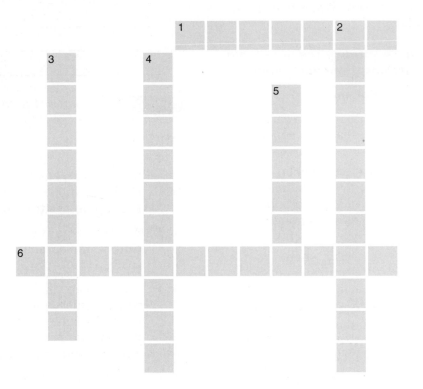

ACROSS

1. This condition occurs when the blood supply to the brain suddenly decreases.

6. This type of shock is caused by a severe allergic reaction (for example, to medications, bee stings, or certain foods, such as nuts).

DOWN

2. Points where the large arteries run close enough to the surface of the skin to be felt as a pulse

3. This is a condition that requires immediate medical or surgical evaluation.

4. This is a condition that is caused by trauma to a blood vessel or by certain illnesses, such as gastric ulcers.

5. This type of shock is caused by severe bacterial infections that involve the entire body.

Activity E *Think About It! Briefly answer the following question in the space provided.*

It is lunch time at Longwood Meadows, the long-term care facility where you work. The residents are eating and talking, when suddenly, Mrs. Lowell, one of the residents, starts to choke and can't seem to get her breath. In the space provided, describe how you would clear Mrs. Lowell's airway.

_____

_____

_____

Activity F *Place an "X" next to the descriptions of people who are at increased risk for choking and aspiration.*

1. _____ People with poorly fitting dentures

2. _____ People with missing teeth

3. _____ Children

4. _____ People who are unconscious, or who have weak coughing or swallowing reflexes

Activity G *Fill in the blanks using the words given in parentheses.*

(syncope, epilepsy, hemorrhage, pulse points, aspiration, abdominal thrusts)

1. _____ is the accidental inhalation of foreign material into the airway.

2. The procedure which is used to clear an obstructed airway in a conscious adult or a child older than 1 year who is choking uses _____ _____.

3. A disorder characterized by chronic seizure activity is called _____.

4. The points where the large arteries run close enough to the surface of the skin to be felt as a pulse are called _____ _____.

5. Severe, uncontrolled bleeding is called _____.

6. _____ is the medical term for fainting.

CHAPTER 14

Assisting With Repositioning and Transferring

ASSISTING WITH REPOSITIONING

Key Learning Points

- Complications caused by immobility
- Six basic body positions
- The words *body alignment, supportive devices, shearing, friction,* and *lift (draw) sheet*

Activity A *Place an "X" next to the reasons for which a person might need to be repositioned.*

1. _____ The person may be in pain.

2. _____ The person may be weak due to an illness or disease.

3. _____ The person may be completely or partially paralyzed.

4. _____ The person may be unconscious or in a coma.

Activity B *A patient who is unable to reposition himself is at risk for developing serious complications. List four complications that can be caused by immobility.*

1. _____

2. _____

3. _____

4. _____

Activity C *Write the name of the body position shown in each of the pictures.*

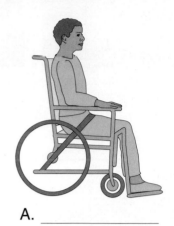

A. _____

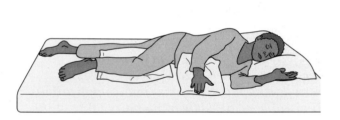

B. _____

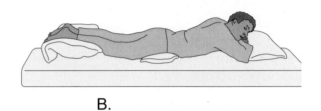

C. _____

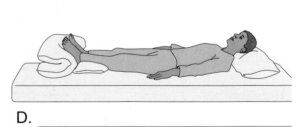

D. _____

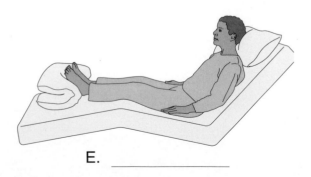

E. _____

Activity D *Match each body position, given in Column A, with its use, given in Column B.*

Column A

_____ **1.** Supine

_____ **2.** Fowler's

_____ **3.** Sims'

_____ **4.** Lateral

Column B

a. Sleeping

b. Relieving pressure on spine

c. Grooming

d. Receiving enema

Activity E *Select the single best answer to the following question.*

1. Which picture below illustrates proper body alignment? _____

A.

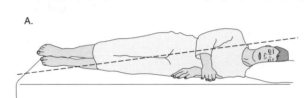

B.

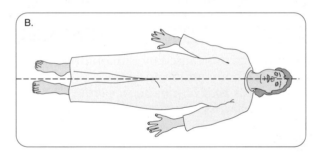

C.

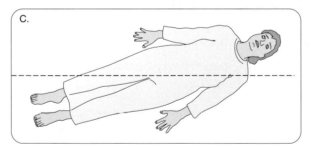

Activity F *Mark each statement as either "true" (T) or "false" (F). Correct the false statements.*

1. **T F** Good body alignment depends on proper body position.

2. **T F** In proper body alignment, an imaginary line runs through the person's nose, breastbone, and pubic bone, and between the person's knees and ankles.

3. **T F** When a person's legs are spread apart, the person is in proper body alignment when each leg is an equal distance from an imaginary line between the two legs.

4. **T F** Proper alignment is not important if a person is placed on his side.

Activity G *Moving a person to the side of the bed is a necessary first step in many procedures. In the spaces below, list 4 measures you can use to help keep your patient or resident and yourself safe while moving the person to the side of the bed.*

1. _____

2. _____

3. _____

4. _____

Activity H *Some of the steps in the procedure for moving a person up in bed are listed here. Write down the correct order of the steps in the boxes provided below.*

1. Have the person bend her knees.

2. Bend your knees slightly to protect your back.

3. Help the person to move smoothly toward the head of the bed.

4. Have the person press her heels to the mattress and lift her buttocks.

5. Place your arm under the person's head and shoulders.

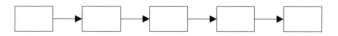

Activity I *Some of the steps in the procedure for turning a person onto his side away from you are listed here. Write down the correct order of the steps in the boxes provided below.*

1. Place one of your hands on the person's shoulder and the other hand on the person's hip nearest you.

2. Bend the person's leg that is nearest you, placing the foot on the bed.

3. Lower the side rail on the working side of the bed.

4. Cross the person's arm that is nearest you over the person's chest.

5. Gently roll the person away from you.

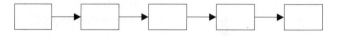

Activity J *Place an "X" next to the statements that are true about logrolling.*

1. _____ Logrolling is done to move a person who has a spinal injury.

2. _____ The person is rolled in one fluid motion and the body is kept in alignment.

3. _____ One assistant is aligned with the person's head and shoulders.

4. _____ The other assistant is aligned with the person's legs.

5. _____ A lift sheet may be used to logroll the person.

6. _____ A pillow is placed lengthwise between the person's legs.

7. _____ The person's arm is folded so that it is on top of his chest when he is turned.

Activity K *Match the words, given in Column A, with their descriptions, given in Column B.*

Column A

_____ **1.** Body alignment

_____ **2.** Supportive devices

_____ **3.** Shearing

_____ **4.** Friction

_____ **5.** Lift (draw) sheet

Column B

a. The force created when something or someone is pulled across a surface that offers resistance

b. A small, flat sheet that is placed over the middle of the bottom sheet, covering the area of the bed from above the person's shoulders to below his or her buttocks

c. Positioning the body so that the spine is not twisted or crooked

d. Devices such as rolled sheets, towels, or blankets used when positioning a person to help the person maintain proper body alignment

e. The force created when two surfaces (such as a sheet and a person's skin) rub against each other

ASSISTING WITH TRANSFERRING

Key Learning Points

- Techniques of safe lifting and transfer
- The terms *transfer, weight-bearing ability,* and *transfer (gait) belt*

Activity A *Think About It! Briefly answer the following question in the space provided.*

A nursing assistant needs to help Mr. Burns transfer from his bed to a wheelchair. Write down four safety measures the nursing assistant should keep in mind when helping Mr. Burns to transfer.

_____

_____

_____

_____

Activity B *Select the single best answer for the following question.*

1. Which of the following devices would you use to help transfer a person to or from a wheelchair safely?

a. A transfer belt

b. A walker

c. Crutches

d. A cane

Activity C *Think About It! Briefly answer the following question in the space provided.*

A patient or resident sitting on the side of the bed is described as "dangling." This is the first step for someone who is getting up from bed to walk. Explain the importance of dangling.

_____

_____

_____

Activity D *Some of the steps in the procedure for transferring a person from a bed to a wheelchair are listed here. Write down the correct order of the steps in the boxes provided below.*

1. Position the person's feet on the footrests of the wheelchair and buckle the wheelchair safety belt. Cover the person's lap with a lap blanket.

2. Help the person put on shoes and a robe, and then apply a transfer belt.

3. Lower the person into the wheelchair by bending your hips and knees.

4. Help the person to move toward the side of the bed, where the wheelchair is located.

5. Lock the wheelchair wheels and swing the footrests to the side.

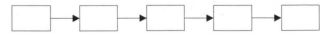

Activity E *Some of the steps in the procedure for transferring a person from a bed to a stretcher are listed here. Write down the correct order of the steps in the boxes provided below.*

1. Raise the level of the bed and lower the head of the bed.

2. Grasp the edge of the lift sheet and roll it over as close to the person's body as possible.

3. Position the lift sheet under the person's shoulders and hips.

4. Position the stretcher alongside the bed and lock the stretcher wheels.

5. Position the person on the stretcher, making sure that her body is in proper body alignment. Buckle the stretcher safety belts across the person and raise the side rails on the stretcher.

6. Ask your three co-workers to lift the person using the lift sheet in unison at the count of three.

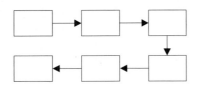

Activity F *Place an "X" next to the statements that are true about using a mechanical lift to transfer a person from the bed to the wheelchair.*

1. _____ Center the sling under the person.

2. _____ The lower edge of the sling should be positioned underneath the person's knees.

3. _____ Spread the legs of the lift to provide a solid base of support.

4. _____ Fasten the sling to the straps of the lift.

5. _____ Allow the person to hold onto the swivel bar.

6. _____ The person faces the wheelchair while being moved with the mechanical lift.

Activity G *Match the words, given in Column A, with their descriptions, given in Column B.*

Column A

_____ 1. Transfer

_____ 2. Weight-bearing ability

_____ 3. Transfer (gait) belt

Column B

a. Assist device used to transfer a person from bed to wheelchair

b. Movement from one place to another (from bed to wheelchair)

c. Ability to stand on one or both legs

Assisting With Exercise

ASSISTING WITH WALKING (AMBULATION)

Key Learning Points

- Benefits of walking
- Assistive devices for walking
- Safety guidelines for assisting a person with walking

Activity A *Place an "X" next to statements that are true about walking.*

1. _____ Helps to improve a person's appetite

2. _____ Prevents constipation

3. _____ Makes a person restless

4. _____ Prevents complications of immobility

5. _____ Is a good form of exercise

Activity B *Place an "X" next to the correct statements for each of the following situations:*

1. Which of the following statements are correct with regard to walking with a walker?

   _____ **a.** The handgrips of the walker should be level with the person's chest.

   _____ **b.** The top of the frame is used for support.

   _____ **c.** The person moves one leg forward and then the other, stepping into the frame of the walker.

   _____ **d.** The tips of the walker are placed flat on the floor.

2. Which of the following statements are correct with regard to walking with a cane?

   _____ **a.** The handle of the cane should be level with the person's hip.

   _____ **b.** The person should hold the cane on the weaker side.

   _____ **c.** All the tips of the cane should be placed flat on the floor at the same time.

   _____ **d.** The nursing assistant should stand slightly behind and to the side on the person's weaker side.

3. Which of the following statements are correct with regard to walking with crutches?

   _____ **a.** The top of the crutches rest underneath the arms of the person.

   _____ **b.** The person supports his weight with his hands on the handgrips.

   _____ **c.** The tips of the crutches are placed flat on the floor.

   _____ **d.** The nurse or physical therapist teaches the person to walk using the crutches.

Activity C *Match the assistive device for walking, given in Column A, with its user, given in Column B.*

Column A

_____ **1.** Walker

_____ **2.** Cane

_____ **3.** Crutches

Column B

a. People who can bear weight but are weak on one side

b. People who cannot bear full weight on one leg

c. People who can bear weight but may be weak or unsteady

Activity D *Mark each statement as either "true" (T) or "false" (F). Correct the false statements.*

1. T F It is important to assist the person to dangle before attempting ambulation.

2. T F Stand behind the person while helping her to stand.

3. T F Stand in front of the person while helping her to walk.

4. T F Assist the person to hold the cane on her strong side.

5. T F A transfer belt may be used if necessary to assist the person to stand up.

6. T F Ensure that the assistive device is in good working order.

Activity E *Place an "X" next to the correct observations in the following situation.*

1. Which of the following observations should be reported to the nurse when assisting a person with walking?

_____ **a.** The person is feeling dizzy and the pulse is weak.

_____ **b.** The person is in pain.

_____ **c.** The person looks pale.

_____ **d.** The person complains of breathlessness.

_____ **e.** The person is breathing normally.

ASSISTING WITH RANGE-OF-MOTION EXERCISES

Key Learning Points

- Benefits of range-of-motion exercises
- Types of range-of-motion exercises
- The word *range of motion*

Activity A *Mark each statement as either "T" true or "F" false. Correct the statements that are false.*

1. T F Normal activities such as dressing, grooming, walking, and eating usually put all of the joints through their complete range of motion.

2. T F The range of motion of a joint is the complete extent of movement that the joint is normally capable of without causing pain.

3. T F Range-of-motion exercises are done to preserve joint and muscle function in a person with limited mobility.

4. T F Regular movement increases aches and pains.

5. T F Range-of-motion exercises may be done while the person is in bed or sitting down.

Activity B *Match the type of range-of-motion exercise, given in Column A, with the amount of assistance needed, given in Column B.*

Column A

_____ **1.** Active range-of-motion exercise

_____ **2.** Active-assistive range-of-motion exercise

_____ **3.** Passive range-of-motion exercise

Column B

a. The nursing assistant helps to complete the movement during exercise.

b. The nursing assistant moves the person's joints through the exercise.

c. The nursing assistant only encourages and directs the person.

Activity C *Fill in the blanks using the words given in parentheses.*

(dorsiflexion, rotation, flexion, pronation, extension, adduction, supination, abduction, inversion, plantar flexion, eversion)

1. _____ involves gentle movement of the head forward, as if to touch the chin to the chest.

2. _____ is the gentle movement of the head backward, with the chin pointing to the sky.

3. The range-of-motion exercise in which the fingers are spread away from each other is called _____.

4. The range-of-motion exercise that involves bringing the fingers back together is called

_____.

5. _____ is turning the hand so that the palm is facing the foot of the bed.

6. _____ is turning the hand so that the palm is facing the head of the bed.

7. _____ is gently bending the foot toward the head.

8. _____ _____ involves gently bending the foot away from the head.

9. _____ exercise involves gently bending the inside of the foot inward.

10. _____ exercise involves gently bending the inside of the foot outward.

11. The range-of-motion exercise involving gentle movement of the head from side to side, as if saying no, is called _____.

Activity D *Select the single best answer for the following question.*

1. When assisting a person with range-of-motion exercises, what should you do?
   a. Follow the care plan or the instructions given to you by the nurse or physical therapist exactly
   b. Move through the exercises in a systematic way
   c. Avoid pushing the joint past its point of resistance
   d. All of the above

CHAPTER 9

Bedmaking

LINENS

Key Learning Points

- Types of linens and their uses
- Handling clean and soiled linens
- The words *bed protector* and *bath blanket*

Activity A *Types of linens used for bedmaking will vary, depending on the type of facility and the needs of the patient or resident. Fill in the blanks using the words given in parentheses.*

(protector, electric, bottom, lift, pillowcase, blanket, moisture, bedspread, mattress, bath)

1. A _____ pad is a thick layer of padding that is placed on the mattress to protect it from moisture and soiling.

2. A _____ sheet is placed over the mattress pad.

3. A _____ sheet is used during repositioning procedures.

4. A bed _____ is used for people who are incontinent or have draining wounds.

5. A _____ may be wool, cotton, or synthetic, depending on the person's preference and the climate.

6. A _____ covers the bed and adds a decorative touch to the person's room.

7. A _____ is used to cover a pillow and protect it from soiling.

8. A _____ blanket is used during bed baths and linen changes.

9. _____ blankets may not be safe to use if the person is incontinent or very young.

10. The lift (draw) sheet also acts as a

    _____ absorbing barrier between the person's body and the mattress if a mattress pad is not being used.

Activity B *Select the single best answer for each of the following questions.*

1. The top sheet used to make a patient's or resident's bed should be:
   a. Fixed
   b. Flat
   c. Fitted
   d. Folded in half

2. An incontinent resident's bed is to be prepared. The nursing assistant uses a rubberized draw sheet to help protect the mattress. What should she place over the rubberized draw sheet to protect the person's skin from contact with the rubber?
   a. A bottom sheet
   b. A moisture-absorbent mattress pad
   c. A cotton lift sheet
   d. A flat sheet

3. How can you provide more efficient and economical care to a patient with a draining wound?
   a. By placing a rubberized sheet next to the person's skin
   b. By using a bed protector

c. By avoiding the use of rubberized or plastic mattresses, which are expensive

d. By covering the wound in such a way that it does not allow the wound to drain

4. Which linen adds a finishing touch to a well-made bed?

a. A top sheet

b. A mattress pad

c. A fitted sheet

d. A bedspread

5. Which of the following linens is not made into the bed?

a. A bed blanket

b. A draw sheet

c. A bath blanket

d. A fitted mattress pad with elasticized sides

Activity C *Think About It! Briefly answer the following question in the space provided.*

Randall is on his way to make up Mr. Walker's bed. What is wrong with this picture?

_____

_____

_____

Activity D *Match the guidelines for bed making, given in Column A, with the reason for their use, given in Column B.*

Column A

_____ 1. Wash your hands before collecting clean linens.

_____ 2. Collect only those linens that you will need for that person's bed.

_____ 3. Collect linens in the order that they will be used.

_____ 4. Wear gloves when removing used linens from a bed.

_____ 5. Place dirty linens in the linen hamper immediately after removing them from the bed.

Column B

a. Helps the facility save extra money and manpower

b. Helps you to remember which linens you need to collect and allows you to make the bed more efficiently

c. Prevents pathogens from being transferred to the clean linens

d. Helps to control the spread of infection from dirty linens

e. Helps to minimize your exposure if the linens are soiled with blood or other body fluids

Activity E *Place an "X" next to each correct answer for the following questions.*

1. Which of the following statements about bed protectors are true?

_____ a. They are used for people who are incontinent.

_____ b. They may be disposable.

_____ c. They are used over a top sheet.

_____ d. They protect the bed from dust when it is not occupied.

_____ e. They are used for people with draining wounds.

2. Which of the following statements about bath blankets are true?

_____ **a.** They are waterproof.

_____ **b.** They are gathered along with the other linens.

_____ **c.** They are used during bed baths.

_____ **d.** They are electric blankets.

_____ **e.** They are used while making an occupied bed.

STANDARD BEDMAKING TECHNIQUES

Key Learning Points

- When a person's linens should be changed
- How to miter a corner
- How to make an occupied bed
- How to make an unoccupied bed
- The words *mitered corner, closed bed, open bed, fanfolded,* and *surgical bed*

Activity A *Place an "X" next to the statements that are true about changing linens.*

1. _____ Routine bed making is usually done in the evening.

2. _____ Linens are changed completely according to the schedule at the facility.

3. _____ The person's bed is remade every time the linens become soiled.

4. _____ An excessively wrinkled bed need not be remade until it is wet or soiled.

5. _____ Routine bed making is usually done in the morning, when the patients or residents are bathing or dressing.

6. _____ Always place linens on the bed so that the seams of the sheets face away from the person's skin.

7. _____ Shake the linens thoroughly before placing them on the bed.

8. _____ Talk reassuringly to the patient while making an occupied bed.

9. _____ Keep the person covered with a bath blanket while making an occupied bed.

10. _____ Check the bed linens for personal items before removing the linens from the bed.

Activity B *The figure shows the steps to make a mitered corner. Look at the following pictures and write down the correct order of the steps.*

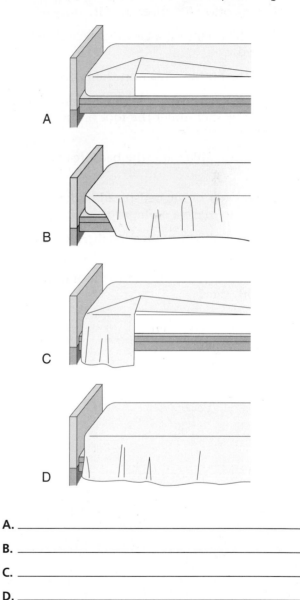

A._____

B._____

C._____

D._____

Activity C *Write down the correct order of steps for making an unoccupied bed in the boxes provided below.*

1. Unfold and center the mattress pad on the bed.

2. Place the top sheet on the bed so that the wide hem will be at the head of the bed.

3. Place a cotton lift sheet over it.

4. Place the linens on a clean surface close to the bed.

5. Place the bottom sheet on the bed.

6. Tuck the bedspread, the blanket, and the top sheet together under the foot of the mattress.

7. Place the blanket and the bedspread on the bed.

8. Fold the top of the bedspread back over the blanket to make a cuff.

9. Place a plastic or rubberized lift sheet over the mattress.

10. Make a mitered corner at the foot of the bed on both sides.

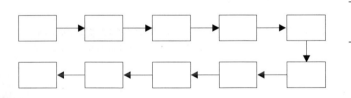

Activity D *Fill in the blanks using the words given in parentheses.*

(occupied, bath blanket, bed bath)

1. When linens are changed while the person is still in the bed, it is called making an

   _____ bed.

2. An occupied bed is generally made after a

   _____ _____.

3. Ensure that the patient or resident is

   covered with a _____ _____
   while making an occupied bed.

Activity E *Match the words, given in Column A, with their definitions, given in Column B.*

Column A	Column B
_____ 1. Surgical bed	a. An empty, made bed
_____ 2. Mitered corner	b. A bed ready to receive a patient or resident
_____ 3. Open bed	c. Top sheet, blanket, and bedspread of a closed bed, turned back
_____ 4. Closed bed	d. A bed ready to receive a patient or resident arriving by stretcher
_____ 5. Fan folded	e. Corners made by folding and tucking the sheet

Measuring and Recording Vital Signs, Height, and Weight

INTRODUCTION TO VITAL SIGNS

Key Learning Points

■ Factors causing changes in a person's vital signs
■ The importance of accurately measuring and recording vital signs
■ The importance of reporting changes in a person's vital signs to the nurse
■ The word *vital signs*

Activity A *Place an "X" next to the factors that can cause a change in a person's vital signs.*

1. _____ Illness

2. _____ Injury

3. _____ Fear

4. _____ Height

5. _____ Pain

6. _____ Anxiety

7. _____ Exercise

8. _____ Profession

Activity B *Mark each statement as either "true" (T) or "false" (F). Correct the false statements.*

1. **T F** Vital signs provide essential information about a person's health.

2. **T F** A major or long-lasting change in a person's vital sign measurements can be a sign of illness.

3. **T F** You should take measurements of vital signs only once, even if measurements are abnormal.

4. **T F** If you are having trouble measuring a patient's or resident's vital signs, you should ask for help from the nurse or another nursing assistant.

Vital signs provide insight into a person's overall health status. Measuring and recording vital signs will be a routine part of your daily duties. Many people are counting on you to provide this information accurately and to report any abnormalities quickly. Your knowledge of your patient or resident will allow you to know whether the vital sign measurements you have obtained are normal readings for the person you are caring for.

Activity C *Fill in the blanks using the words given in parentheses.*

(subjective, recording, objective, nursing care, reporting, nurse)

1. It is the duty of a nursing assistant to routinely measure and record a person's vital signs

   and promptly report to the _____ if abnormal changes are detected.

2. The _____ _____ plan will provide the nursing assistant with information regarding the routine measurement of each patient's or resident's vital signs.

3. Vital sign measurements are called

   _____ data.

4. _____ data include the patient's or resident's complaint of pain, dizziness, or nausea.

5. Measuring,_____, and _____ vital sign measurements accurately is critical because this information is used to make important decisions about the patient's or resident's care.

Activity D *Place an "X" next to the statements that are true about vital signs.*

1. _____ They provide essential information about a person's health.

2. _____ Body temperature, pulse, respirations, and blood pressure are vital signs.

3. _____ The normal range for vital signs is the same for everybody.

4. _____ Measuring, reporting, and recording vital sign measurements accurately is critical.

5. _____ Vital sign measurements are used to make important decisions about the patient's or resident's care.

BODY TEMPERATURE

Key Learning Points

- Common sites for measuring body temperature
- Normal range for an adult's temperature
- How to use a glass thermometer and an electronic thermometer

- How to measure an oral, rectal, axillary, and tympanic temperature
- The word *fever*

Activity A *Match the types of temperatures, given in Column A, with the quality that best describes them, given in Column B.*

Column A	Column B
_____ 1. Oral temperature	a. Slow and least accurate measurement
_____ 2. Rectal temperature	b. Obtained from the person's forehead
_____ 3. Axillary temperature	c. Cannot be taken if the person has an injury in the mouth
_____ 4. Tympanic temperature	d. Very accurate but can be embarrassing for the person
_____ 5. Temporal temperature	e. Taken in the ear

Activity B *Mark each statement as either "true" (T) or "false" (F). Correct the false statements.*

1. **T F** The normal oral temperature for an adult ranges from 36.5°C to 37.5°C.

2. **T F** A temperature higher than normal could be a sign of illness or infection.

3. **T F** It is not necessary to report a slight increase or decrease in an elderly person's temperature.

4. **T F** The normal temporal temperature is 98.6°F.

5. **T F** The method used to measure the temperature affects the accuracy of the measurement, so it is important to note which method was used when you recorded the temperature.

Activity C *Fill in the blanks using the words given in parentheses.*

1. The mercury in a glass thermometer must

   be "shaken down" to below the _____ (94° mark/100° mark) on a Fahrenheit thermometer or the 34° mark on a Celsius thermometer.

2. The glass thermometer is washed with

_____ (warm/hot) water and soap.

3. The glass thermometer is rinsed with cool

water, and placed in a _____ (disinfectant/medicated) solution.

4. The disinfectant solution is _____ (rinsed/wiped) off the glass thermometer before use.

5. To read the temperature on a glass

thermometer, hold it _____ (vertically/horizontally) by the stem at eye level.

6. Rotate the glass thermometer until the line of

_____ (mercury/ink) becomes visible.

7. Record the temperature at the end of the line

_____ _____ (farthest away from/ nearest to) the bulb in a glass thermometer.

8. When using an/a _____ (electronic/ glass) thermometer, a probe is placed in the patient's or resident's mouth, rectum, or armpit to measure the temperature.

9. Before use, the probe of an electronic

thermometer is covered with a _____ (disposable/permanent) sheath.

10. The temperature is displayed on a screen

on the _____ (front/side) of the electronic thermometer.

Activity D *Place an "X" next to each correct answer for the following questions.*

1. Which of the following precautions should be taken when measuring an oral temperature?

_____ **a.** If the person has eaten, consumed a beverage, chewed gum, or smoked within the last 15 minutes, wait for another 15 to 30 minutes before taking the oral temperature.

_____ **b.** It is safe to use a glass thermometer even if it has a slight crack.

_____ **c.** The end of the glass thermometer or an electronic probe should be covered with a disposable sheath before use.

_____ **d.** The temperature reading should be indicated with an "O" when you record it.

2. Which of the following precautions should be taken when measuring a rectal temperature?

_____ **a.** Lubricate the tip of the thermometer to ease insertion.

_____ **b.** Leave the person alone after the thermometer is inserted.

_____ **c.** Do not force the thermometer into the rectum.

_____ **d.** Do not insert the thermometer more than 1 inch for an adult or 1/2 inch for a child.

3. Which of the following statements are true about measuring an axillary temperature?

_____ **a.** You can measure a person's axillary temperature 5 minutes after the person has had a bath or applied deodorant or antiperspirant.

_____ **b.** Pat the axilla (underarm area) with a paper towel before positioning the thermometer.

_____ **c.** A glass thermometer should be kept in position for 10 minutes or according to facility policy before reading the temperature.

_____ **d.** The temperature reading should be indicated with an "A" when you record it.

4. Which of the following precautions should be taken when measuring a tympanic temperature?

_____ **a.** If the person wears a hearing aid, remove it and take the person's temperature immediately.

_____ **b.** Excessive ear wax should be wiped off with a warm, moist washcloth.

_____ **c.** The covered probe should be pointing down and toward the front of the ear canal.

_____ **d.** The temperature reading should be indicated with a "T" when you record it.

Activity E *Place an "X" next to statements that are true for fever.*

1. _____ It is a sign of illness or infection.

2. _____ It is a body temperature between 97.6°F and 99.6°F.

3. _____ It is a body temperature of more than 37.5°C.

4. _____ It should be reported to the nurse immediately.

PULSE

Key Learning Points

- Qualities to be noted when taking a person's pulse
- Common sites used for taking a person's pulse
- The proper way to measure and record a radial pulse and an apical pulse
- The normal range for an adult's pulse rate
- The words *pulse rate, pulse rhythm, pulse amplitude, stethoscope,* and *pulse deficit*

Activity A *Mark each statement as either "true" (T) or "false" (F). Correct the false statements.*

1. T F The normal adult heart rate is between 60 and 100 beats per minute.

2. T F A weak or thready pulse usually means that the heart is having trouble circulating blood throughout the body.

3. T F Normally, the time between each pulsation varies.

4. T F Each pulsation should be strong and easy to feel.

5. T F Any change in pulse rate, rhythm, or amplitude should be reported to the nurse immediately.

Activity B *Fill in the blanks using the words given in parentheses.*

(radial, skin, pulse, carotid, apical)

1. The _____ reflects the rate, rhythm, and strength of the heartbeat.

2. The pulse is a throbbing sensation just underneath the _____ .

3. The pulse can be felt by placing your fingers gently over the _____ artery in the neck.

4. The pulse can be felt by placing your fingers gently over the _____ artery in the wrist.

5. The _____ pulse is measured by listening over the apex of the heart with a stethoscope.

Activity C *Place an "X" next to the statements that are true about taking a person's radial pulse.*

1. _____ The thumb should be placed over the radial artery to count the number of pulses.

2. _____ The middle two or three fingers should be placed over the radial artery to count the number of pulses that occur in either 30 seconds or 1 minute.

3. _____ Although the pulse may be taken at other pulse points, taking the pulse at the radial artery is easiest for the patient or resident.

4. _____ The radial pulse is a common way of measuring the pulse rate.

Activity D *You have been asked to measure a person's apical pulse using a stethoscope. Look at the following pictures and write down the correct order of the steps.*

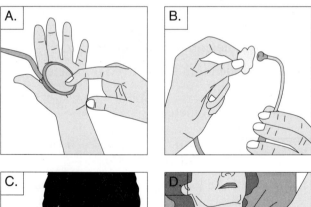

A. _____

B. _____

C. _____

D. _____

Activity E *Match the words, given in Column A, with their definitions, given in Column B.*

Column A

_____ **1.** Pulse rate

_____ **2.** Pulse rhythm

_____ **3.** Pulse amplitude

_____ **4.** Stethoscope

_____ **5.** Pulse deficit

Column B

a. A device that amplifies sound and transfers it to the listener's ears

b. The difference between the apical pulse rate and the radial pulse rate

c. The pattern of pulsations and the pauses between them

d. The number of pulsations that can be felt over an artery in 1 minute

e. The force or quality of the pulse

RESPIRATION

Key Learning Points

- Qualities to be noted when measuring a person's respirations
- The proper way to measure and record a person's respirations
- The normal range for an adult's respiratory rate
- The words *respiratory rate, respiratory rhythm, depth of respiration,* and *dyspnea*

Activity A *Fill in the blanks using the words given in parentheses.*

(exhale, breathing, respiratory rhythm, depth of respiration, inhale, respiratory rate)

1. Respiration is the process of _____.

2. The chest rises each time we _____

and falls each time we _____.

3. By looking at and counting a person's respirations, we are able to tell the

_____ _____ _____,

_____ _____, and

_____ _____.

Activity B *Place an "X" next to the statements that are correct.*

1. _____ Counting respirations can be done by looking at the person's chest.

2. _____ Counting respirations can be done by placing your hand near the collarbone or on the person's side.

3. _____ Each rise and fall of the chest is one respiration.

4. _____ If the respiratory rhythm is irregular, count the number of breaths that occur in 30 seconds.

5. _____ If the respiratory rhythm is regular, count the number of breaths that occur in 60 seconds.

Activity C *Mark each statement as either "true" (T) or "false" (F). Correct the false statements.*

1. T F The normal adult respiratory rate is between 10 and 15 beats per minute.

2. T F The chest should rise and fall in a regular rhythm.

3. T F Breathing should be quiet and easy.

4. T F Any change in respiratory rate, rhythm, or depth should be reported to the nurse immediately.

Activity D *Match the words, given in Column A, with their definitions, given in Column B.*

Column A

_____ **1.** Respiratory rate

_____ **2.** Respiratory rhythm

_____ **3.** Depth of respiration

_____ **4.** Dyspnea

Column B

a. The regularity with which a person breathes

b. Labored or difficult breathing

c. The number of times a person breathes in 1 minute

d. The quality of each breath

BLOOD PRESSURE

Key Learning Points

- The parts of a sphygmomanometer
- The normal range for an adult's blood pressure
- The words *systolic pressure, diastolic pressure, sphygmomanometer, hypertension, hypotension,* and *orthostatic hypotension*

Activity A *Some of the steps in the procedure for taking a person's blood pressure are listed below. Write down the correct order of the steps in the boxes below.*

A. Place the stethoscope over the brachial artery and inflate the cuff slowly until the pulse can be heard through it.

B. Continue to inflate the cuff until the pulse cannot be heard.

C. Pump the bulb to inflate the cuff.

D. Wrap the cuff around the person's upper arm where the brachial artery is located.

E. Turn the valve on the bulb slightly counterclockwise to allow air to escape from the cuff slowly.

F. Continue to inflate the cuff 30 mm Hg more.

G. Note the reading on the manometer when the first sound of the pulse is heard.

H. Place the diaphragm of the stethoscope directly over brachial artery and close the valve on the bulb by turning it clockwise.

I. Continue to deflate the cuff and note the reading on the manometer when the last sound of the pulse is heard.

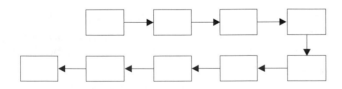

Activity B *Match the parts of a sphygmomanometer, given in Column A, with their descriptions, given in Column B.*

Column A	Column B
_____ 1. Cuff	a. A gauge that measures the air pressure in the cuff
_____ 2. Bulb	b. A flat, cloth-covered inflatable pouch, wrapped around the person's upper arm
_____ 3. Manometer	c. Squeezed or pumped to fill the cuff with air

Activity C *Mark each statement as either "true" (T) or "false" (F). Correct the false statements.*

1. **T F** The accepted normal range for the diastolic pressure is between 100 and 140 mm Hg.

2. **T F** The accepted normal range for the systolic pressure is between 60 and 90 mm Hg.

3. **T F** Blood pressure readings are usually lowest in the morning.

4. **T F** Blood pressure readings are usually slightly higher after a meal.

5. **T F** If one of your patients or residents who has been diagnosed with hypertension is not taking his medicine as ordered, you should report this to the nurse immediately.

Activity D *Fill in the blanks using the words given in parentheses.*

(hypotension, diastolic, systolic, orthostatic, hypertension, sphygmomanometer)

1. The pressure that the blood exerts against the arterial walls when the heart muscle contracts is called _____ pressure.

2. A _____ is a device used to measure blood pressure.

3. A blood pressure that is consistently greater than 140 mm Hg (systolic) and/or 90 mm Hg (diastolic) is called _____.

4. The pressure that the blood exerts against the arterial walls when the heart muscle relaxes is called _____ pressure.

5. A blood pressure that is consistently lower than 90 mm Hg (systolic) and/or 60 mm Hg (diastolic) is called _____.

6. A sudden decrease in blood pressure that occurs when a person stands up from a sitting or lying position is called _____ hypotension.

Activity E *Look at the pictures below. The readings on the manometer for all "A" figures are systolic pressures and for all "B" figures are diastolic pressures. Write the pressure readings for each pair and specify whether the reading falls within the range of normal.*

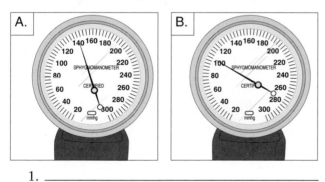

1. _____

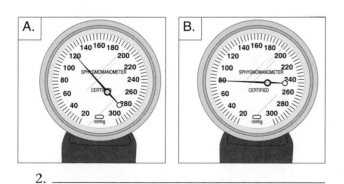

2. _____

HEIGHT AND WEIGHT

Key Learning Points

- Why measuring a person's weight accurately is important
- The proper way to measure a person's height and weight using an upright scale
- The proper way to measure a person's weight using a chair scale

Activity A *Place an "X" next to the statements that are true.*

1. _____ Changes in weight allow the health care team to evaluate the person's nutritional status.

2. _____ Changes in weight can give information about how well a person's heart and kidneys are working.

3. _____ Changes in weight can indicate disease.

4. _____ Some medications are prescribed according to body weight.

5. _____ It is important to measure height each time weight is measured.

6. _____ Height and weight measurements are obtained as frequently as vital sign measurements.

Activity B *Write down the correct order of the steps for measuring height and weight using an upright scale in the boxes provided below.*

1. Adjust the height bar until it just touches the person's head.

2. Ask the person to urinate.

3. Allow the person to stand on the scale platform without holding on to anything.

4. Move weights all the way to the left of the balance bar.

5. Note the height and weight of the person.

6. Move the weights on the scale bar until the balance pointer is centered between the two scale bars.

7. Report a change in weight to the nurse.

8. Hold the height rod and help the person to step down from the scale.

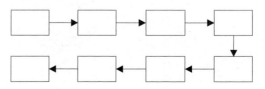

Activity C *Look at the figures below and write down the weight measurement shown on each.*

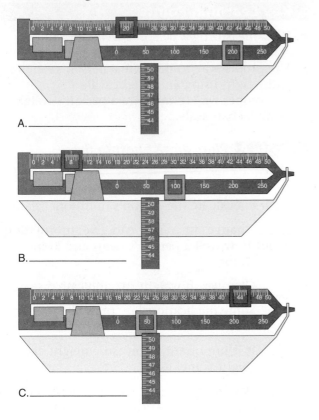

A. _____

B. _____

C. _____

Activity D *Think About It! Briefly answer the following question in the space provided.*

1. The nurse has asked you to obtain the height and weight of several residents. How will you do it?

   a. Ms. Quinlan is in a coma.

   _____

   b. Mrs. Lorenz cannot stand for a very long

   period of time. _____

   c. Mr. Pepper is able to get out of bed and

   walk with help. _____

Assisting With Hygiene

INTRODUCTION TO PERSONAL HYGIENE

Key Learning Points

- The importance of good personal hygiene
- Scheduling of routine care
- The word *PRN (as-needed) care*

Activity A *List three benefits of good personal hygiene.*

1. _____

2. _____

3. _____

Activity B *Following are routine activities associated with personal hygiene that are performed at different times during the day. Place an "EM" next to activities that are a part of early morning care, an "M" next to activities that are a part of morning care, an "A" next to activities that are part of afternoon care, and an "E" next to activities that are part of evening (hs, hour of sleep) care.*

1. _____ General housekeeping duties, such as tidying the person's room and changing the bed linens

2. _____ Straightening the bed linens

3. _____ A general "freshening up" involving assistance with using the toilet, washing of the hands and face, and oral care

4. _____ Preparing the person for breakfast or early diagnostic testing or treatment

5. _____ Helping the person to change into pajamas

6. _____ Assisting with insertion of dentures prior to eating breakfast

7. _____ Assisting with using the toilet, bathing, oral care, shaving, hair care, dressing, and putting on make-up

Activity C *Select the single best answer for the following question.*

1. When is PRN (as-needed) care given?
   a. According to the schedule in the person's nursing care plan
   b. Whenever there is wetness or soiling of the skin, clothing, or bedding
   c. When the doctor orders it
   d. When there is time to provide it

⬤ Make an effort to accommodate your patients' or residents' individual requests with regard to when personal hygiene activities are carried out whenever possible. Also, remember: people with wet or soiled skin, linens, or clothing require immediate attention!

ASSISTING WITH ORAL CARE

Key Learning Points

- The benefits of good oral hygiene
- How to assist with oral hygiene
- The frequency of oral hygiene

Activity A *Place an "X" next to the statements that are true.*

1. _____ Poor oral hygiene can cause gum disease and bad breath.

2. _____ Brushing teeth thoroughly can lead to dental cavities and tooth loss.

3. _____ A clean mouth feels good and makes food taste better.

4. _____ Good oral hygiene contributes to overall health.

Activity B *Place an "X" next to the observations that you should immediately report to the nurse when assisting a patient or resident with oral hygiene.*

1. _____ Dry, red, cracked, or bleeding lips

2. _____ Loose or broken teeth

3. _____ Minty-smelling breath

4. _____ Fruity-smelling breath

5. _____ A clean tongue

6. _____ Poorly fitting dentures

Activity C *Mark each statement as either "true" (T) or "false" (F). Correct the false statements.*

1. **T F** Routine oral care is usually provided every 2 hours.

2. **T F** People who are unable or not allowed to take food or fluids by mouth will need oral care every 1 or 2 hours.

3. **T F** People who are taking medications that cause a dry mouth will need oral care every 1 or 2 hours.

Activity D *Fill in the blanks using the words given in parentheses.*

(lukewarm, dentures, dry, solution, washcloth)

1. _____ take the place of a person's natural teeth, allowing the person to chew his or her food properly.

2. Dentures should be stored in a denture cup filled with _____ water.

3. Denture _____ prevents the dentures from drying out and warping.

4. Placing the dentures inside the mouth is more difficult when the mouth is

_____.

5. When cleaning dentures, line the sink with a

_____ or paper towels.

Activity E *Some of the steps for assisting a person to brush her teeth are listed below. Write down the correct order of the steps in the boxes provided below.*

A. Wet the toothbrush. Put a small amount of toothpaste on the toothbrush.

B. Gather your supplies and cover the over-bed table with paper towels.

C. Offer the person the cup of water and ask her to rinse her mouth completely.

D. Brush the tongue.

E. Raise the head of the bed as tolerated. Place a towel under the person's chin.

F. Hold the emesis basin underneath the person's chin so that she can spit the water into the basin.

G. Position the toothbrush at a 45-degree angle to the gums, and move gently in a circular motion.

H. Dry the person's mouth and chin thoroughly using a towel.

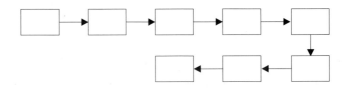

A clean, healthy mouth makes food taste better, provides a line of defense against infection, and allows a person to chew food properly.

Activity F *Select the single best answer for each of the following questions.*

1. Mrs. Jones wears dentures. What should you do when assisting Mrs. Jones with oral care?
   a. Dry the dentures before placing them in her mouth.
   b. Rinse her mouth with water or mouthwash and use a soft toothbrush or a sponge-tipped swab to clean her gums, tongue, and the insides of the cheeks.
   c. Place the dentures in a denture cup and cover them with hot water.
   d. Write Mrs. Jones' name and age on the denture cup.

2. Where do you place dentures when cleaning them?
   a. In a sink lined with a washcloth
   b. In the patient's or resident's mouth
   c. In the palm of your hand
   d. On the counter or over-bed table

Activity G *Think About It! Briefly answer the following question in the space provided.*

One of your residents, Mr. Brentwood, is in a coma. When providing oral care for Mr. Brentwood, why do you turn his head to the side? What is the purpose of using a padded tongue blade when providing oral care to Mr. Brentwood?

_____

_____

_____

_____

Activity H *Select the single best answer for the following question.*

1. A person is said to be edentulous if
   a. He has a broken tooth
   b. He is wearing dentures
   c. He has cavities
   d. He is without teeth

ASSISTING WITH PERINEAL CARE

Key Learning Points

- Why perineal care is an essential aspect of daily hygiene
- Observations that need to be reported to the nurse with regard to perineal care
- Sensitivity issues that a nursing assistant should be aware of when assisting with perineal care
- The proper technique for providing perineal care
- The word *perineal care (peri-care)*

Activity A *Select the single best answer for each of the following questions.*

1. Why is good perineal care important?
   a. It prevents infection, skin breakdown, and odor
   b. It prevents bad breath
   c. It helps the patient or resident to remain independent
   d. All of the above

2. Which of the following can cause skin breakdown and odor in the perineal area?
   a. Irritants on the skin, such as feces, urine, and menstrual blood
   b. Use of a soapless cleanser
   c. An unwillingness to shave the private area
   d. Not being circumcised

3. Which of the following should be done when providing perineal care?
   a. Rinse away all soap and dry the skin thoroughly.
   b. Ask the person's consent for the procedure before beginning.
   c. Take standard precautions.
   d. All of the above

Activity B *Place an "X" next to the observations that should be reported to the nurse when assisting a patient or resident with perineal care.*

1. _____ Abnormal odor
2. _____ Unusual redness, inflammation, or skin rashes in the perineal area

3. _____ Bleeding from the vagina in a postmenopausal woman

4. _____ Bleeding from the anus

5. _____ Lack of pain during menstruation

Activity C *Think About It! Briefly answer the following question in the space provided.*

Assisting a patient or resident with perineal care can be embarrassing for both the patient or resident and the nursing assistant. Write down how you would handle each of the following potentially embarrassing situations.

1. You have to provide perineal care for a member of the opposite sex.

_____

_____

_____

2. A male patient or resident becomes sexually aroused while you are providing perineal care.

_____

_____

_____

Activity D *Fill in the blanks using the words given in parentheses.*

(circular, circumcision, retract)

1. _____ is a procedure involving the removal of the foreskin, the fold of loose skin that covers the head of the penis.

2. If the person is circumcised, place your washcloth covered hand at the tip of the

penis and wash in a _____ motion, downward to the base of the penis.

3. If the person is uncircumcised, _____ the foreskin and clean the area using a different part of the washcloth each time, until the area is clean.

Activity E *Mark each statement as either "true" (T) or "false" (F). Correct the false statements.*

1. T F When providing perineal care, spread the bath blanket over the person and fanfold the top linens to the foot of the bed.

2. T F When providing female perineal care, make sure to wipe from the anal area upwards toward the vulva.

3. T F Use a different washcloth for cleaning each side of the vulva and the middle until the area is clean.

4. T F Always wash toward the anus.

Activity F *Select the single best answer for the following question.*

1. What is perineal care?

   a. Cleaning the anus

   b. Cleaning the perineum and anus, as well as the vulva (in women) and the penis (in men)

   c. Cleaning the area between the bottom of the vagina and the anus in women and the root of the penis and the anus in men

   d. Cleaning the penis in men and the vulva in women

ASSISTING WITH BATHING

Key Learning Points

- The benefits of bathing
- Observations that a nursing assistant should make while assisting a person with bathing and skin care
- Supplies used for bathing
- Sensitivity issues that a nursing assistant should be aware of when assisting with bathing
- Safety issues related to assisting with a tub bath or shower
- The proper technique for assisting a patient or resident with a tub bath or shower
- The proper technique for assisting a patient or resident with a bed bath

Activity A *Place an "X" next to the correct answers for the following questions.*

1. Which of the following are benefits of a bath?

   _____ a. Makes the person feel relaxed and refreshed

   _____ b. Eliminates bad breath

   _____ c. Exercises muscles that might otherwise not be used

   _____ d. Stimulates blood flow to the skin

_____ **e.** Helps the person meet cultural and religious needs

_____ **f.** Gives the nursing assistant an opportunity to observe skin problems

_____ **g.** Reduces the risk of infection

2. Which of the following observations should you report to the nurse when assisting a patient or a resident with bathing?

_____ **a.** New rashes, bruises, broken skin, bleeding, or unusual odors

_____ **b.** Red, pale, or bluish skin

_____ **c.** A flaking, itchy, or sore scalp or the presence of nits

_____ **d.** New hair loss (anywhere on the body)

Activity B *Match the skin care products, given in Column A, with their descriptions, given in Column B.*

Column A

_____ **1.** Soapless cleanser

_____ **2.** Bath oil

_____ **3.** Lotion or cream

_____ **4.** Body powder

_____ **5.** Deodorant or antiperspirant

Column B

a. Prevents perspiration and body odor

b. Prevents drying and chapping

c. Perfumes bath water and moistens skin

d. May not need to be rinsed away; often used to clean the perineal area

e. Absorbs sweat and reduces friction between skin

Activity C *Mark each statement as either "true" (T) or "false" (F). Correct the false statements.*

1. T F   Always explain to the person how the bathing procedure will be carried out before starting the procedure.

2. T F   Always keep the bathroom door locked during the procedure.

3. T F   When assisting the person to and from the bathroom, make sure that he is adequately covered.

4. T F   Gather all necessary equipment, linens, bath products, and clothing during the bath.

Activity D *You are getting ready to assist Mr. Granger with a tub bath. Write down the correct order of the steps in the boxes provided below.*

A. Assist Mr. Granger with undressing.

B. Ask Mr. Granger if he needs to use the toilet.

C. Assist Mr. Granger out of the bath and onto a towel-covered chair.

D. Fill the tub with warm water at the proper temperature.

E. Assist Mr. Granger with washing his face.

F. Assist Mr. Granger with perineal care.

G. Assist Mr. Granger to the tub room.

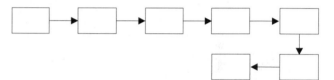

Allowing people to participate in their own self-care helps to maintain independence, but assisting as necessary helps to ensure that hygiene is performed thoroughly.

Activity E *Select the single best answer for each of the following questions.*

1. Which one of the following is an acceptable temperature for a tub bath?

   a. 110°F

   b. 98.6°F

   c. 125°F

   d. 212°F

2. When assisting a person with a tub bath or shower, which of the following should you do?

   a. Place a nonskid mat on the floor of the tub or shower

   b. Take standard precautions

   c. Leave the door unlocked

   d. All of the above

3. When giving a bed bath, when is the water in the basin changed?

   a. After washing each body part

   b. Whenever the water becomes cool or soapy

   c. Only if the resident requests fresh water

   d. Only before bathing the next resident

4. When giving a person a bed bath, where is the bath blanket placed?

   a. Under the person

   b. Under the top linens

   c. Over the top linens

   d. Under the wash basin

19

Preventing Pressure Ulcers and Assisting With Wound Care

PREVENTING PRESSURE ULCERS

Key Learning Points

- How pressure ulcers form
- Conditions that increase a person's risk for developing a pressure ulcer
- Why prevention of pressure ulcers is important
- Changes in the skin that could be signs of a pressure ulcer
- How nursing assistants help to prevent pressure ulcers
- Special equipment used to prevent pressure ulcers
- The words *pressure ulcer* and *pressure points*

Activity A *Place an "X" next to the conditions that can lead to the development of a pressure ulcer.*

1. _____ Part of a person's body presses against a surface, such as a mattress

2. _____ A person sleeps on wrinkled bed linens

3. _____ A person sits on a bedpan for a long period

4. _____ A person wears a splint or brace that presses against the skin

5. _____ A person has a rash

Activity B *Some of the events that lead to the development of a pressure ulcer are listed below. Write down the correct order of the steps in the boxes provided below.*

1. Tissue death occurs as a result of a lack of oxygen.

2. The tissues do not receive enough nutrients and oxygen.

3. Pressure squeezes the tissue between the bone and the surface the person is resting on.

4. The dead tissue peels off or breaks open, creating an open sore.

5. Blood flow to the tissues decreases.

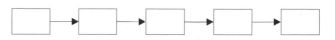

Activity C *The four stages of a developing pressure ulcer are shown on the next page. Look at the pictures and write down the correct order of the stages in the boxes provided below them.*

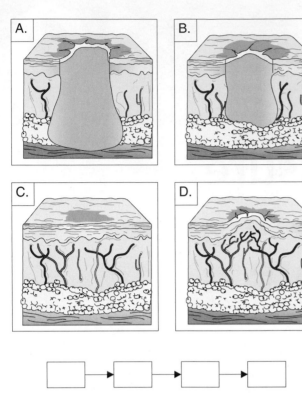

Activity E *Match the risk factors, given in Column A, with the reason they put a person at risk for a pressure ulcer, given in Column B.*

Column A

_____ **1.** Old age

_____ **2.** Poor nutrition and inadequate fluid intake

_____ **3.** Prolonged contact with water

_____ **4.** Cardiovascular problems

_____ **5.** Friction and shearing injuries

Column B

a. Skin does not have what it needs to remain healthy

b. Skin is injured, leading to skin breakdown

c. Skin becomes fragile and thin, with less blood flow

d. Epidermis softens and breaks down

e. Tissues do not receive full amount of oxygen and nutrients

Activity D *Look at the figures and mark the pressure points where pressure ulcers are likely to form.*

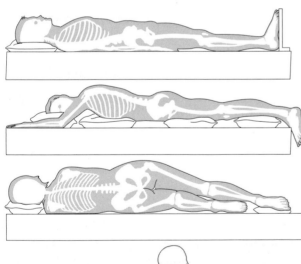

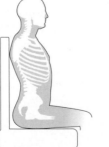

Activity F *Mark each statement as either "true" (T) or "false" (F). Correct the false statements.*

1. T F One of the criteria used to evaluate the quality of care given by long-term care facilities that receive government funding is the health care team's ability to prevent residents from getting pressure ulcers.

2. T F The nurse is not responsible for assessing each resident's risk for developing pressure ulcers when the resident is admitted to the long-term care facility.

3. T F The nurse documents any existing pressure ulcers for all residents.

4. T F Pressure ulcers are not painful, but are difficult to treat.

5. T F Pressure ulcers can cause a person to die.

Activity G *As a nursing assistant, there are many things you can do to help keep a person's skin healthy. Briefly describe what the nursing assistant is doing to keep the person's skin healthy in each of the figures below.*

D. _____

E. _____

F. _____

G. _____

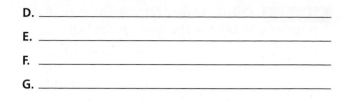

You will do many things to prevent your patients or residents from developing pressure ulcers, including repositioning, observing, providing good skin and perineal care, changing wet and soiled linens promptly, and encouraging exercise.

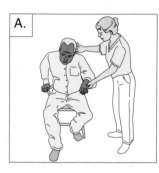

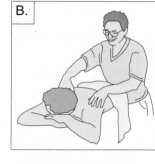

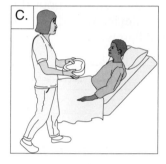

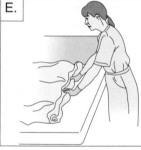

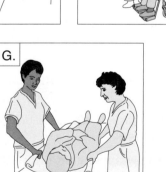

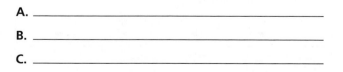

Activity H *Match the pieces of equipment used to prevent pressure ulcers, given in Column A, with their descriptions, given in Column B.*

Column A

_____ 1. Bed board

_____ 2. Elbow pads and heel booties

_____ 3. Footboard

_____ 4. Pressure-relieving mattress

_____ 5. Bed cradle

Column B

a. Used to keep the top sheet, blanket, and bed-spread off the patient's or resident's feet

b. A sheet of wood placed under the mattress to provide extra support

c. A padded board placed upright at the foot of the bed

d. Placed on top of the regular mattress to help prevent skin breakdown

e. Helps to prevent the skin from rubbing against sheets or other surfaces

A. _____

B. _____

C. _____

Activity I *Think About It! Briefly answer the following question in the space provided.*

Mr. Vincente, a home health care client, is 72 years old. He has congestive heart failure. Because it is difficult for him to walk and he tires very easily, Mr. Vincente usually moves from the bed to his easy chair in front of the television in the morning and stays there all day, getting up only occasionally to go to the bathroom. Because Mr. Vincente is a widower and he doesn't have much interest in cooking, he eats mostly microwave dinners and prepackaged snacks. Mr. Vicente lives in the southern United States, where it gets very hot and humid in the summer, and his house is not air-conditioned. What risk factors for the development of a pressure ulcer does Mr. Vincente have?

_____

_____

_____

ASSISTING WITH WOUND CARE

Key Learning Points

- Observations that a nursing assistant may make related to wound care that should be reported to the nurse
- Proper technique for assisting with a dressing change
- The word *wound*

Activity A *Fill in the blanks using the words given in parentheses.*

(drains, dressings, drainage, wound, skin)

1. The _____ is the body's first line of defense against infection.

2. A _____ creates an opening that allows microbes to enter the body, putting the person at risk for infection.

3. As part of the healing process, some wounds produce a lot of fluid, also known as

_____.

4. Wound _____ may be used to remove fluids from the wound.

5. _____ are applied to wounds to prevent microbes from gaining access to the body, to keep the wound dry, or to absorb drainage from the wound.

Activity B *Place an "X" next to the conditions that can delay wound healing.*

1. _____ Multiple injuries

2. _____ Young, healthy patient

3. _____ Weakened immune system

4. _____ Poor nutrition

5. _____ Fluid in the wound

Activity C *Think About It! Briefly answer the following question in the space provided.*

You are caring for Mr. Smith, who has a wound drain that is connected to a collection device. You know that you should check the collection device frequently. What observations about the drainage in the collection device would you report to the nurse immediately?

_____

_____

_____

Activity D *Listed below are some of the steps in the procedure for assisting a nurse with a dressing change. Write down the correct order of the steps in the boxes provided below.*

A. Help the person to a comfortable position that allows access to the wound.

B. If the nurse asks you to, take the old dressing from the nurse and place it in the cuffed plastic bag.

C. If the nurse asks you to, secure the dressing by placing one piece of tape along each side of the dressing.

D. Position the bed at a comfortable working height.

E. Put on a mask, a gown, or both if necessary. Put on gloves.

F. Open the wrapper containing the dressing and hold it open.

G. Remove your gloves and dispose of them. Put on a clean pair of gloves.

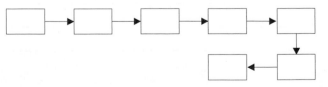

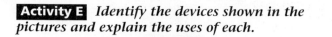
Activity E   *Identify the devices shown in the pictures and explain the uses of each.*

1.

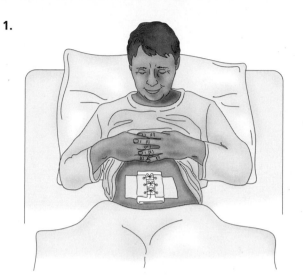

_____

_____

_____

3.

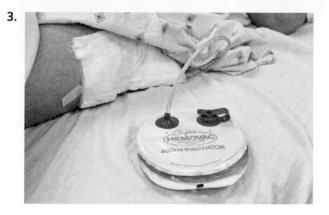

_____

_____

_____

2.

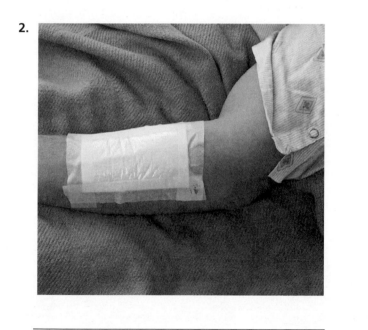

_____

_____

_____

Assisting With Grooming

INTRODUCTION TO GROOMING

Key Learning Points

- The importance of respecting a person's preferences with regard to grooming habits whenever possible
- The importance of assisting a person with grooming

Activity A *Place an "X" next to the activities that are considered "grooming" activities.*

1. _____ Shampooing and styling the hair

2. _____ Bedmaking

3. _____ Applying make-up

4. _____ Providing nail care

5. _____ Assisting with exercise

6. _____ Shaving

Activity B *Think About It! Briefly answer the following question in the space provided.*

1. List three factors that can influence a person's grooming practices.

_____

_____

_____

Activity C *Think About It! Briefly answer the following question in the space provided.*

You have been assigned to care for Mr. Robert. You are quite surprised when Mr. Robert tells you he is expecting visitors and asks you if you would be willing to help him apply his make-up. How would you respond, and why?

_____

_____

_____

ASSISTING WITH HAND CARE

Key Learning Points

- The importance of proper hand care
- Observations that should be reported when assisting a patient or resident with hand care
- The technique for assisting with hand care
- The word *hangnails*

Activity A *Select the single best answer for each of the following questions.*

1. Which of the following are signs of good health that might be observed when providing nail care?

   a. The nail beds are pink.

   b. There is no gap between the nail and the nail beds.

c. The cuticles are smooth and unbroken.

d. All of the above

2. Which statement regarding nail care is true for a disoriented or comatose person?

a. A disoriented or comatose person is not aware of his fingernails' length or appearance, so it is not important to provide nail care for him.

b. A disoriented or comatose person is more likely to have hangnails and fungal infection of the nails.

c. A disoriented or comatose person's fingernails should be kept smooth and short.

d. It is best to provide nail care for a person who is disoriented or comatose when the nails are hard and dry.

3. When is the best time to perform nail care?

a. At least 2 hours before a meal

b. At least 2 hours following a bath

c. During or immediately following a bath

d. There is no ideal time for this activity

Activity B *Fill in the blank with the correct word.*

1. _____ are broken pieces of cuticle that cause injury and pain.

ASSISTING WITH FOOT CARE

Key Learning Points

- Changes that occur in a person's feet as a result of aging or illness
- Observations that should be reported when assisting a patient or resident with foot care
- The technique for assisting with foot care
- The word *podiatrist*

Activity A

Mrs. McAndrews has diabetes. What sorts of changes would you inspect her feet for, while you are assisting her with foot care? Why is being observant for changes in the feet of a person with diabetes especially important?

_____

_____

_____

Activity B *Select the single best answer for each of the following questions.*

1. When caring for a person's feet, you should do all of the following EXCEPT:

a. Soften the nails by soaking them for a short time in warm water

b. Trim or file corns or calluses

c. File the nails so that the edges are smooth

d. Apply foot powder or lotion to the feet after they are dry

2. What type of health care professional specializes in care of the feet?

a. The nurse

b. The nursing assistant

c. The doctor

d. The podiatrist

3. An elderly person's toenails are usually:

a. Soft and flexible

b. Ingrown

c. Yellow, hard, and thick

d. Easy to trim

Activity C *Use the clues to complete the crossword puzzle.*

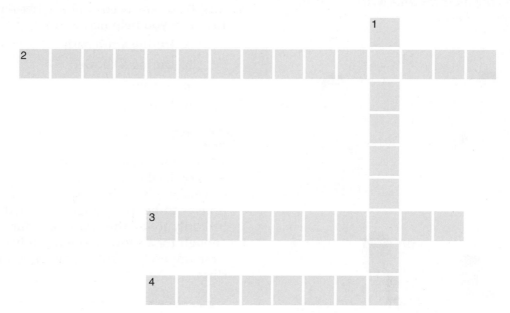

ACROSS

2. A condition where the nail curves down and back into the skin, causing injury and pain

3. A doctor who specializes in the care of the feet

4. A tool used to trim nails

DOWN

1. Broken pieces of cuticle skin, causing injury and pain

ASSISTING WITH DRESSING AND UNDRESSING

Key Learning Points

- The technique for assisting a person who has a weak arm or leg or an intravenous (IV) line to dress
- The technique for assisting a person with dressing
- The technique for changing a hospital gown

Activity A *Mark the statements as either "true" (T) or "false"(F). Correct the false statements.*

1. **T F** When assisting a person to dress or undress, you should first disconnect the person's IV line.

2. **T F** When helping a person with a paralyzed arm or leg to dress, you should place the garment's sleeve or leg onto the paralyzed arm or leg first.

3. **T F** While assisting a patient with a hospital gown, put on gloves if contact with broken skin is likely.

Activity B *Place an "X" next to the statements that are true about helping a person to dress.*

1. _____ All patients and residents wear the same clothing, per facility policy.

2. _____ Allowing a person to choose the clothing he or she wishes to wear is a top priority when assisting with dressing.

3. _____ Patients and residents are used to dressing and undressing in the presence of others.

4. _____ The type of clothing a person wears will differ according to the person's abilities.

Activity C *A person who has an intravenous (IV) line in place needs your help to dress. Look at the following pictures and write down the correct order of the steps.*

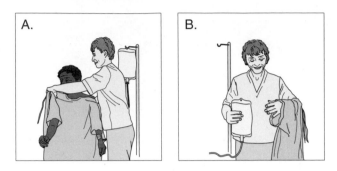

A.

B.

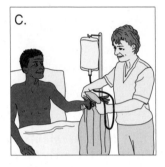

C.

A. _____

B. _____

C. _____

Activity D *Mrs. Colins needs assistance in order to undress. She is wearing a dress that fastens in the back. Briefly describe how you will help Mrs. Colins undress.*

_____

_____

_____

ASSISTING WITH HAIR CARE

Key Learning Points

- Methods used to assist a person with shampooing the hair
- The technique for shampooing a person's hair in bed
- The technique for combing a person's hair
- Methods used to style a person's hair
- Observations that should be reported when assisting a person with hair care

Activity A *Place an "X" next to the correct answers.*

1. Mrs. Bradshaw needs to have her hair washed. How can you help her do this?

_____ a. During a tub bath

_____ b. During a shower

_____ c. At the sink

_____ d. In bed, using a shampoo trough

Activity B

The doctor has ordered complete bed rest for Ms. Loyd, who is 7 months pregnant with triplets and is in the hospital due to complications with her pregnancy. Ms. Loyd leaves bed only to use the bathroom, but not long enough for a shower. The nurse has asked you to shampoo Ms. Loyd's hair. How will you do this?

_____

_____

_____

Activity C *Mark the statements as either "true" (T) or "false" (F). Correct the false statements.*

1. T F If a person's hair is matted or tangled, it may need to be cut.

2. T F It is not necessary to ask a person's permission before cutting his or her hair.

3. T F To remove tangles from the hair, use a wide-tooth comb and start at the scalp, working down to the ends of the hair.

Activity D *Identify what is wrong with the following picture.*

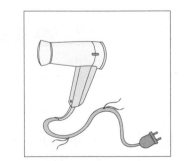

_____

_____

_____

ASSISTING WITH SHAVING

Key Learning Points

- The importance of shaving as a routine grooming practice for both men and women
- The technique for assisting a person to shave

Activity A *Mark the statement as either "true" (T) or "false" (F). Correct the statement if it is false.*

1. **T F** Beards and mustaches must be kept clean and free of food and drink, and they must be trimmed and brushed regularly.

Activity B *Select the single best answer to the following question.*

1. You notice that Mr. Smith's razor blade has become very dull, and you replace it. How should you dispose of the old razor blade?

    a. Dispose of it in a facility-approved waste container.

    b. Dispose of it in a sharps container.

    c. Leave it on Mr. Smith's over-bed table; the housekeeping staff will dispose of it.

    d. Take it to the nurses' station.

Activity C *Mr. Flanders needs his face shaved. Some of the steps in the procedure for shaving a man's face are listed below. Write down the correct order of the steps in the boxes provided below.*

A. Shave the area between Mr. Flanders' nose and upper lip.

B. Place a towel across Mr. Flanders' shoulders and chest.

C. Fill the wash basin with warm water.

D. Shave Mr. Flanders' chin.

E. Apply shaving cream, gel, or soap to the beard.

F. Shave Mr. Flanders' neck.

G. Shave Mr. Flanders' cheeks.

H. Apply aftershave lotion, if Mr. Flanders requests it.

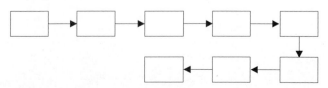

Activity D *Mrs. Robinson asks you to shave her armpits. Briefly describe how you would do this.*

_____

_____

_____

ASSISTING WITH VISION AND HEARING ACCESSORIES

Key Learning Points

- Caring for eyeglasses
- Caring for contact lenses
- Caring for prosthetic (artificial) eyes
- Caring for a person's hearing aid
- The technique for inserting and removing an in-the-ear hearing aid

Activity A *The following sentences are related to helping a person care for eyeglasses, contact lenses, or an artificial eye. Fill in the blanks using the words given in parentheses.*

(contact lens, prosthetic eye, solutions, eyeglasses)

a. Clean _____ with a cloth and a special solution made specifically for that purpose, or with warm water.

b. A _____ is made of molded plastic and fits directly on the eyeball.

c. The types of _____ that are used with contact lenses vary according to the type of lens.

d. A person who has had an eye removed may choose to wear a _____, which is made of ceramic or plastic and is usually designed to be very close in appearance to the person's own eye.

Activity B *Mark the statements as either "true" (T) or "false" (F). Correct the false statements.*

1. **T F** Contact lenses should be cleaned and soaked in tap water.

2. **T F** Hearing aids must not be exposed to extreme heat or cold, moisture, or hairspray.

3. **T   F**   Improper handling can lead to nicks and scratches on prosthetic eyes.

4. **T   F**   Hearing aids need to removed and cleaned weekly.

Activity C   *Mr. Williams needs help inserting his in-the-ear hearing aid. Write down the correct order of the steps in the boxes provided below.*

A. Turn on the control switch and adjust the volume by talking to Mr. Williams as you increase the volume. Stop when he can hear you.

B. Inspect the hearing aid, to check for cracks and proper battery insertion.

C. Inspect the ear canal for excessive wax.

D. Help Mr. Williams into a comfortable position.

E. Make sure the hearing aid is turned off and the volume is low.

F. Repeat for the other ear if required.

G. Gently insert the tapered end into the ear canal. Rotate gently. Push up and in, gently pulling down on the earlobe. See that the hearing aid fits snugly and comfortably.

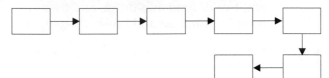

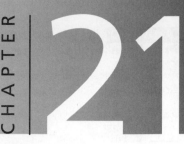
Assisting With Nutrition

INTRODUCTION TO NUTRITION

Key Learning Points

- General types of nutrients
- What is considered a healthy diet
- The words *nutrition, nutrients, calories,* and *glucose*

Activity A *Select the single best answer for each of the following questions.*

1. What is nutrition?
   a. The process of breaking down food into simple elements
   b. An essential element of food
   c. The unit of energy released by food inside our bodies
   d. The process of taking in and using food

2. Which of the following nutrients regulates body processes?
   a. Fats
   b. Minerals
   c. Proteins
   d. Carbohydrates

3. How do proteins help our bodies?
   a. They protect our organs and help us stay warm.
   b. They rebuild tissues that break down from normal use or as a result of illness or injury.
   c. They help regulate body processes.
   d. They help prevent constipation.

Activity B *Match the words, given in Column A, with their definitions, given in Column B.*

Column A

_____ 1. Ingestion

_____ 2. Digestion

_____ 3. Absorption

_____ 4. Metabolism

Column B

a. The breaking down of foods into simple elements

b. The transfer of nutrients from the digestive tract into the bloodstream

c. The conversion of nutrients into energy in cells

d. The intake of food

Activity C *Mark each statement as either "true" (T) or "false" (F). Correct the false statements.*

1. T F The energy to power our bodies comes from water.

2. T F Protein is found in foods such as milk and cheese, meat, poultry, fish, eggs, nuts, and dried peas and beans.

3. T F Extra carbohydrates that are not used immediately as fuel are either stored in the liver or converted to fat and stored elsewhere in the body.

Activity D *Match the type of nutrient, given in Column A, with its description, given in Column B.*

Column A

_____ 1. Water

_____ 2. Fat

_____ 3. Minerals

_____ 4. Vitamins

_____ 5. Carbohydrates

Column B

a. Helps to regulate body processes

b. Provides no calories or nutritional value but is essential to life

c. Provides structure within the body and regulates body processes

d. Protects our organs and helps us to stay warm

e. The source of the body's most basic type of fuel, glucose

Activity E *Fill in the blanks using the words given in parentheses.*

(fruit, vegetables, milk, meat and beans, grain)

1. Eat at least 3 oz of whole- _____ cereals, breads, crackers, rice or pasta every day.

2. Choose fresh, frozen, canned, or dried _____ and be sure to eat 2 cups every day.

3. Eat 2½ cups of _____ every day, including carrots, sweet potatoes, spinach, and broccoli.

4. _____ are a good source of protein; be sure to choose low-fat or lean sources.

5. Go low-fat or fat-free when you choose _____, yogurt, and other dairy products.

FACTORS THAT AFFECT FOOD CHOICES AND EATING HABITS

Key Learning Points

■ Factors that influence a person's food preferences

■ OBRA regulations related to meals in long-term care facilities

■ The words *appetite* and *anorexia*

Activity A *Think About It! Briefly answer the following question in the space provided.*

Many factors influence the choices we make about food every day. List five factors that influence your food choices, and give an example of each from your own personal experience.

_____

_____

Activity B *Long-term care facilities that receive government funding must follow Omnibus Budget Reconciliation Act (OBRA) regulations pertaining to meals. Fill in the blanks below using the words given in parentheses.*

(attractive, individual, preference, religious, others, proper, health)

1. OBRA requires that meals meet the _____ nutritional needs of each resident.

2. Foods must be served at the _____ temperature.

3. Meals must be _____ to look at and seasoned to the individual resident's

_____.

4. Special diets, such as those followed for _____ or _____ reasons must be provided for those residents who need them.

5. Dining in the company of _____ is also recommended.

Activity C *Fill in the blanks using the words given in parentheses.*

(anorexia, appetite)

1. Mrs. Tibbs tells you she just doesn't have any interest in eating anymore, since her husband died. Mrs. Tibbs is suffering

from _____.

2. Mr. McEldowney has been smelling dinner cooking all day, and he is very hungry.

Mr. McEldowney has an _____.

SPECIAL DIETS

Key Learning Points

- Common special diets
- The words *dietitian* and *nutritional supplement*

Activity A *Match the type of diet, given in Column A, with its description, given in Column B.*

Column A	Column B
_____ 1. Regular "house" diet	a. Low in fats
_____ 2. Clear liquid diet	b. Regulates the amount of fat, carbohydrate, and protein
_____ 3. Full liquid diet	c. A small amount of salt may be allowed, or none at all
_____ 4. Soft diet	d. Well-balanced diet with no restrictions on specific foods or condiments
_____ 5. Diabetic diet	e. Clear liquids, plus foods that can be poured at room or body temperature
_____ 6. Sodium-restricted diet	f. Most foods are chopped or creamed
_____ 7. Low cholesterol diet	g. Foods that can be poured at room temperature and that you can see through

Activity B *Mark each statement as either "true" (T) or "false" (F). Correct the false statements.*

1. **T F** Foods that are considered clear liquids include milk, vanilla ice cream, and juice.

2. **T F** A person on a sodium-restricted diet is not allowed to have salt at all.

3. **T F** Nutritional supplements are used to replace meals.

4. **T F** A dietitian has a degree in nutrition.

Taking the time to learn about a person's medical condition and the reason a particular diet was ordered will make you a more effective member of the health care team.

ASSISTING WITH MEALS

Key Learning Points

- The importance of making meals attractive and the dining experience pleasant
- How to prepare a person for meal time
- Ways to help a person during meal time
- Proper technique for feeding a person who cannot feed herself
- How to record the amount of solid food eaten
- Observations to report when assisting a person to eat

Activity A *Think About It! Briefly answer the following question in the space provided.*

Many patients and residents have little or no appetite. List five things that can decrease a person's appetite. Then, list five things you can do to help increase a person's appetite.

_____

_____

_____

_____

_____

_____

Activity B *Place an "X" next to the type of assistance a nursing assistant may be expected to provide at meal time.*

1. _____ Removing the cover from the tray

2. _____ Describing the foods and their location on the tray to the person

3. _____ Seasoning food according to your taste

4. _____ Serving dessert only when the person has eaten all of the main course

5. _____ Turning on the radio or television for the person to enjoy

6. _____ Giving the person his medication

Activity C *Think About It! Briefly answer the following question in the space provided.*

After dinner, you notice that Mrs. Li did not touch her soup but ate all the noodles that you had served. Why should you talk about why she did not eat her soup? Write down what you would say to Mrs. Li to begin the conversation.

_____

_____

_____

_____

Activity D *Select the single best answer for the following question.*

1. What should you do while feeding a dependent patient or resident?

   a. Remain standing while feeding the person, for good body mechanics

   b. Use a fork to feed the person

   c. Give the person enough time to chew and swallow each bite

   d. Offer liquids sparingly

Activity E *You are assisting Mrs. Giamelli, who has poor eyesight, with eating her dinner. You know that if you describe the location of the food in terms of a clock face, Mrs. Giamelli will be able to eat fairly well on her own. Fill in the numbers on the clock face shown below and then write down how you would describe the location of the food on the plate to Mrs. Giamelli.*

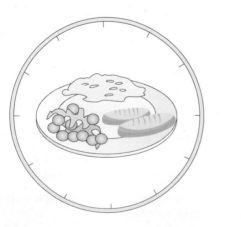

_____

_____

Activity F *It is dinnertime at the long-term care facility and you are assisting Mr. Linkins with his meal. Some of the steps that are taken when assisting a person with a meal are given below. Write down the correct order of the steps in the boxes provided below.*

1. Ask Mr. Linkins if he would like to use a clothing protector.

2. Check the meal tray to make sure that it has Mr. Linkins' name on it and that it contains the correct diet for Mr. Linkins.

3. Wash Mr. Linkins' hands and face.

4. Assist Mr. Linkins with toileting.

5. Uncover the meal tray and tell Mr. Linkins what is on the tray.

6. Allow Mr. Linkins to assist with the eating process to the best of his ability.

7. Remove the tray and the clothing protector, if used.

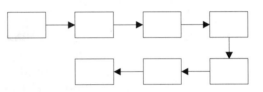

Activity G *The nurse has asked you to record the percentage of each food that Mr. Flannery eats during the meal. Mr. Flannery's meal tray before and after dinner is shown below. Record your answers.*

1. _____ Chicken

2. _____ Mashed potatoes

3. _____ Salad

4. _____ Ice cream

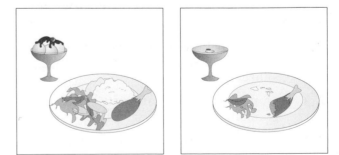

Activity H *Mark each statement as either "true" (T) or "false" (F). Correct the false statements.*

1. T F Wearing a clothing protector is a matter of personal choice so it is important to ask the resident if he wants to wear a clothing protector or not.

2. T F When assisting a person with a meal, it is important not to talk.

3. T F Assistive devices, such as specially made eating utensils, help a disabled person regain independence, which is important for self esteem.

⬤ When our emotional needs are met, it is easier for us to meet our physical needs. Ensuring that mealtime is pleasant can help improve a person's appetite.

ASSISTING WITH FLUIDS

Key Learning Points

- The importance of water for life
- Factors affecting fluid balance
- How to measure and record a person's fluid intake
- Fluids that are considered "output"
- The words *fluid balance, edema, NPO status,* and *graduate*

Activity A *Mark each statement as either "true" (T) or "false" (F). Correct the false statements.*

1. T F Water forms the basis for many important body fluids.

2. T F Water intake is essential for life.

3. T F Edema is too little fluid in body tissue.

4. T F Only those taking medications suffer from dehydration.

Activity B *Match the body fluids, given in Column A, with their descriptions, given in Column B.*

Column A

_____ **1.** Cytoplasm

_____ **2.** Plasma

_____ **3.** Urine

_____ **4.** Sweat

_____ **5.** Mucus

_____ **6.** Synovial fluid

Column B

a. Liquid part of blood

b. Helps to keep the body cool

c. Jelly-like substance inside the body's cells

d. Helps our joints to move smoothly

e. Keeps the mucous membranes moist

f. Carries waste products out of the body

Activity C *Mark each statement as either "true" (T) or "false" (F). Correct the false statements.*

1. T F Encouraging fluid intake involves offering small amounts of a drink frequently throughout the day.

2. T F Before surgery or a diagnostic procedure, a patient or resident may be placed on NPO status.

3. T F People generally complain of "dry mouth" when their fluid intake is restricted.

4. T F A person on NPO status is not allowed to consume any kind of fluids.

Activity D *Match the words, given in Column A, with their definitions, given in Column B.*

Column A

_____ 1. Dehydration

_____ 2. NPO status

_____ 3. Graduate

_____ 4. Edema

_____ 5. Fluid balance

Column B

a. A doctor's order for some patients or residents prior to surgery or a diagnostic procedure

b. Too much fluid in the tissues of the body

c. A measuring device used to measure fluids

d. A state where the amount of fluid taken into the body equals the amount of fluid that leaves the body

e. Too little fluid in the tissues of the body

Activity E *Think About It! Briefly answer the following questions in the spaces provided.*

1. You have been asked to calculate fluid intake of the following residents. Write down the fluid intake of each resident in milliliters.

   a. Mr. Scott's meal tray contained a 12-ounce can of soda, an 8-ounce carton of milk, and 120 mL of water at the beginning of the meal. He finished his soda and milk but drank only half of the water.

   _____

   b. Ms. Sean's tray contained an 8-ounce glass of orange juice, 240 mL of coffee, and one 6-ounce container of ice cream. She drank half of the juice and all of the coffee, and she ate half the container of ice cream.

   _____

   c. Mr. Ray's tray contained a 16-ounce glass of iced tea, an 8-ounce carton of milk, and 180 mL of broth. He drank three-fourths of the glass of tea and all of his milk, but no broth.

   _____

Activity F *List five fluids that are considered "output."*

1. _____
2. _____
3. _____
4. _____
5. _____

ALTERNATE METHODS OF PROVIDING NUTRITION AND FLUIDS

Key Learning Points

- Conditions that may make an intravenous (IV) line necessary
- Observations that should be reported when caring for a person with an IV line
- Ways of providing nutrition to people who are unable to take food by mouth
- Observations that should be reported when caring for a person receiving IV fluids or enteral nutrition
- The word *enteral nutrition*

Activity A *Fill in the blanks using the words given in parentheses.*

(intravenous therapy, enteral nutrition, regurgitation, infusion pump)

1. To help avoid _____ and aspiration, the head of the bed is raised during enteral feeding.

2. _____ is used to give fluids through a person's blood vessels.

3. Enteral feedings may be given at scheduled times or continuously by an _____.

4. _____ involves placing food directly into the stomach or intestines, which eliminates the need for the person to chew or swallow.

Activity B *Descriptions of some feeding tubes are given below. The names of those feeding tubes are listed in jumbled form. Use the pictures and descriptions as clues to form the correct words.*

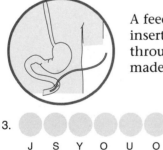

A feeding tube that is inserted through the nose, down the throat, and into the stomach.

1. ◯◯◯◯◯◯◯◯◯◯◯
A T C A N S I O R S G

A feeding tube that is inserted into the stomach through a surgical incision made in the abdomen.

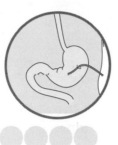

2. ◯◯◯◯◯◯◯◯◯◯◯
R S M G T Y A O S O T

A feeding tube that is inserted into the jejunum through a surgical incision made in the abdomen.

3. ◯◯◯◯◯◯◯◯◯◯◯
J S Y O U O E M T N J

Activity C *Think About It! Briefly answer the following question in the space provided.*

Mr. Nash has an IV line. List 6 things to check for when caring for Mr. Nash.

1. _____

2. _____

3. _____

4. _____

5. _____

6. _____

CHAPTER 22

Assisting With Urinary Elimination

INTRODUCTION TO URINARY ELIMINATION

Key Learning Points

- How the urinary system removes waste products from the body
- The characteristics of normal urine
- Observations that should be reported when assisting a person with urinary elimination
- Actions that promote normal urinary elimination
- The words *urination, micturition, voiding, hematuria, frequency, urgency, nocturia,* and *dysuria*

Activity A *Fill in the blanks using the words given in parentheses.*

(urethra, kidneys, bladder, ureters)

1. Blood passes through the ___Kidneys___, which remove waste products and excess fluid, forming urine.

2. Urine flows from the kidneys through the ___ureters___ and is stored in the urinary bladder.

3. As the ___bladder___ fills, we begin to feel the urge to urinate.

4. Urine leaves the body through the ___urethra___.

Activity B *Place an "X" next to the characteristics of normal urine.*

1. _____ Clear without cloudiness or particles

2. _____ Slight red tinge

3. _____ Pale yellow, straw-colored, or dark gold (amber) in color

4. _____ A very strong ammonia smell

5. _____ May become cloudy as it cools

Activity C *Mark each statement as either "true" (T) or "false" (F). Correct the false statements.*

1. (T) F Urine with a slight odor should be reported to the nurse.

2. (T) F The nurse should be informed if the person complaints of pain or burning during urination.

3. (T) F Cloudy or bloody urine should be reported to the nurse.

4. (T) F Urine with an unusual odor or appearance could be a sign of illness or infection.

5. T (F) A change in voiding habits or new episodes of incontinence do not need to be reported to the nurse.

Activity D *Make a list of at least five things you can do to help promote normal urinary elimination for your patients or residents.*

1. _____
2. _____
3. _____
4. _____
5. _____

Activity E *Fill in the blanks using the words given in parentheses.*

(frequency, micturition, dysuria, hematuria, nocturia, urgency, voiding)

1. The process of passing urine from the body is called urination, or _Micturition_, or _Voiding_.

2. A slight red tinge to the urine may indicate _Hematuria_.

3. Urination that occurs more often than usual is called _Frequency_.

4. The need to urinate immediately is called _Urgency_.

5. The need to get up more than once or twice during the night to urinate, to the point where sleep is disrupted, is called _Nocturia_.

6. A person having painful or difficult urination is said to have _Dysuria_.

ASSISTING WITH BEDSIDE COMMODES, BEDPANS, AND URINALS

Key Learning Points

- Equipment used to assist people with urinary elimination
- How to assist a person with a bedpan
- How to assist a person with a urinal
- The words *bedside commode, bedpan, fracture pan,* and *urinal*

Activity A *Mark each statement as either "true" (T) or "false" (F). Correct the false statements.*

1. T (F) The patient or resident who cannot get out of bed uses a bedside commode.

2. (T) F Handrails are attached alongside the toilet to make it easier for the person to sit down and get back up.

3. (T) F Men who cannot get out of bed use a urinal for elimination of urine.

4. (T) F Devices for obtaining urine specimens include a specimen container, a commode hat, a bedpan, and a urinal.

5. (T) F Standard precautions should be taken when assisting a person with urination.

Activity B *Place an "X" next to the statements that are true when assisting a person with a bedpan.*

1. _X_ Bedpans can bruise or tear the fragile skin of an elderly or disabled person.

2. _____ A person with back injuries or a hip fracture can use the standard bedpan.

3. _X_ A fracture pan is positioned with the narrow end pointed toward the head of the bed.

4. _X_ If the person is on intake and output status, the urine output should be measured and recorded.

5. _X_ If the person's condition allows, raise the head of the bed to promote a more natural elimination position.

Activity C *Match the equipment, given in Column A, to its use, given in Column B.*

Column A	Column B
_c_ 1. Bedside commode	a. A device used when a person is unable to get out of bed
_a_ 2. Bedpan	b. A device used for urination when a man is unable to get out of bed
_d_ 3. Fracture pan	c. A chairlike frame with a toilet seat and a removable collection bucket used when a person is able to get out of bed, but unable to walk to the bathroom
_b_ 4. Urinal	

d. A wedge-shaped bedpan that is used when a person has a back injury or hip fracture

3. (T) F The end of the tubing should be wiped with an antibacterial wipe before reconnecting the urine drainage bag.

4. T (F) The urine drainage bag can be attached to the side rail of the bed.

CARING FOR A PERSON WITH AN INDWELLING URINARY CATHETER

Key Learning Points

- Conditions that may make use of an indwelling urinary catheter necessary
- How to handle the catheter tubing and urine drainage bag
- How to provide routine urinary catheter care
- How to empty a urine drainage bag
- Observations that should be reported when caring for a person with an indwelling urinary catheter
- The words *catheter* and *catheter care*

Activity A *Place an "X" next to the conditions that may make use of an indwelling urinary catheter necessary.*

1. X____ The person is very ill, weak, or disabled, and is unable to urinate using a toilet, bedpan, urinal, or bedside commode.

2. ____ The person is incontinent of urine and inserting a catheter will be more convenient for the staff.

3. X____ The person's bladder needs to be emptied before or after a surgical procedure.

4. X____ The person is incontinent of urine and has wounds or pressure ulcers that would be made worse by contact with urine.

5. ____ The person has a urinary tract infection.

6. X____ The person cannot remember to call for assistance when he or she needs to use the bathroom.

Activity B *Mark each statement as either "true" (T) or "false" (F). Correct the false statements.*

1. (T) F The catheter tubing is secured to the person near the insertion site.

2. T (F) The urine drainage bag is secured at a level higher than the bladder.

Activity C *Fill in the blanks using the words given in parentheses.*

(health care–associated, vulva, mitt, circular, urethra)

1. Form a __mitt__ around your hand with a washcloth.

2. Rinse and dry the __vulva__ and perineum thoroughly in a woman with a catheter.

3. Retract the foreskin, clean the tip of the penis. and wash in a __circular__ motion toward the base of the penis.

4. Hold the catheter near the opening of the __urethra__ to prevent tugging on the catheter as you clean it.

5. Catheter care is done to reduce the risk of a __HAI__ infection.

Activity D *Place an "X" next to the statements that are true for emptying urine drainage bags.*

1. ____ "Leg bags" need to be emptied more frequently because they hold less urine.

2. X____ Urine is drained into a graduate.

3. ____ The emptying spout is cleaned with water after the urine has been drained.

4. X____ If the person is on intake and output status, measure the urine.

5. ____ Unusual observations about the urine should be reported to the doctor.

Activity E *Make a list of five observations that need to be reported when caring for a person with an indwelling urinary catheter.*

1. _____

2. _____

3. _____

4. _____

5. _____

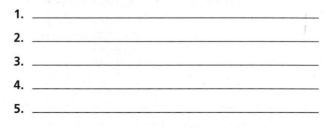

Activity F *Fill in the blanks using the words given in parentheses.*

(perineal, health care–associated, catheter)

1. A tube that is inserted into the body for the purpose of administering or removing fluids is called a ___Catheter___.

2. Catheter care involves thorough cleaning of the ___perineal___ area and the catheter tubing that extends outside of the body, to prevent infection.

3. Catheter care is done to reduce the risk of ___HAI___ infection in people with indwelling urinary catheters.

CARING FOR A PERSON WHO IS INCONTINENT OF URINE

Key Learning Points

- Common types of urinary incontinence
- Physical and emotional effects of urinary incontinence
- Products that are used to manage urinary incontinence
- Bladder training
- The words *urinary incontinence, urinary retention,* and *condom catheter*

Activity A *Match the type of urinary incontinence, given in Column A, with its description, given in Column B.*

Column A	Column B
_C_ 1. Stress incontinence	a. Occurs when the bladder is too full of urine
_e_ 2. Urge incontinence	b. Occurs in the absence of physical or nervous system problems affecting the urinary tract
_b_ 3. Functional incontinence	
_a_ 4. Overflow incontinence	c. Occurs when the person coughs, sneezes, or exerts herself
_d_ 5. Reflex incontinence	

d. Occurs when there is damage to the nerves that allow the person to control urination

e. Occurs in cases of urinary tract infection

Activity B

1. List two ways in which urinary incontinence can affect a person physically.

    a. _____

    b. _____

2. List two ways in which urinary incontinence can affect a person emotionally.

    a. _____

    b. _____

Activity C *Place an "X" next to the statements that are true.*

1. _X_ Incontinence pads are placed on the bed to keep the bed linens dry.

2. _X_ Incontinence briefs may be worn instead of regular underpants.

3. _X_ Bed protectors are placed on the bed to keep the bed linens and mattress dry.

4. _X_ A condom catheter consists of a soft plastic or rubber sheath placed over the penis and a collection bag attached to the leg.

Activity D *Fill in the blanks using the words given in parentheses.*

(incontinent, scheduling, involuntary)

1. ___Scheduling___ helps promote regular emptying of the bladder.

2. Bladder training is commonly used to help people who are ___incontinent___ of urine.

3. The main goal of bladder training is for the person to be able to control ___involuntary___ urination.

Activity E *Match the words, given in Column A, with their definitions, given in Column B.*

Column A

_c_ **1.** Urinary incontinence

_a_ **2.** Urinary retention

_b_ **3.** Condom catheter

Column B

a. The inability of the bladder to empty either completely during urination, or at all

b. A device used to manage urinary incontinence in men

c. The involuntary loss of urine from the bladder

OBTAINING A URINE SPECIMEN

Key Learning Points

- Proper technique for collecting a routine urine specimen
- Proper technique for collecting a midstream ("clean catch") urine specimen
- The words *urinalysis* and *midstream ("clean catch") urine specimen*

Activity A *Mark each statement as either "true" (T) or "false" (F). Correct the false statements.*

1. T (F) When a midstream ("clean catch") urine specimen is needed, the person is asked to urinate directly into the specimen container.

2. (T) F When a routine urine specimen is needed, the person may urinate into a specimen collection device.

3. T (F) If the person has a bowel movement during the urine specimen collection, it will not affect the results.

4. T (F) Toilet paper can be placed in the collection device.

5. (T) F Urine is poured from the specimen collection device into the specimen container.

Activity B *Select the single best answer for the following question.*

1. Which statement is true about collecting a midstream ("clean catch") urine specimen?

   a. A bedpan is used to collect the urine specimen.

   b. Perineal care is provided before the sample is collected.

   c. The person begins to urinate, then stops, then starts again, and the urine sample is collected from the restarted flow.

MEASURING URINE OUTPUT

Key Learning Points

- Methods used to measure and record urine output
- The words *oliguria, polyuria, diuresis,* and *anuria*

Activity A *Fill in the blanks using the words given in parentheses.*

(kidneys, urine output, commode hat, flow sheets, graduate, fluid, markings)

1. _Urine Output_ is simply the amount of urine the person voids over a given period of time.

2. A person's urine output gives information regarding the functioning of a person's _Kidneys_.

3. Urine output can help to tell us whether or not the person is maintaining a good _Fluid_ balance.

4. The person may be asked to void into a _Commode hat_ (a specimen collection device) to measure his urine output.

5. Urine output can be measured by pouring it into a _graduate_.

6. Specimen collection devices, urinals, and the drainage bags used with urinary catheters often have _Markers_ that make measuring urine output easy.

7. Intake and output (I&O) _Flow_ _Sheet_ will have spaces to record the amount of each individual voiding.

Activity B *Solve the crossword puzzle, using the clues given below.*

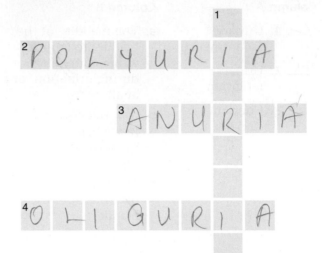

ACROSS

2. Another term for "diuresis"

3. The state of voiding less than 100 mL of urine over the course of 24 hours

4. The state of voiding only 100 to 400 mL of urine over 24 hours over a given period of time

DOWN

1. Excessive urine output

Assisting With Bowel Elimination

INTRODUCTION TO BOWEL ELIMINATION

Key Learning Points

- How the digestive system removes waste products from the body
- The characteristics of normal feces
- How to promote normal bowel elimination
- The words *chyme* and *defecate*

Activity A *Fill in the blanks using the words given in parentheses.*

(enzymes, bloodstream, stomach, feces)

1. The food is broken down in the _____.

2. The food is mixed with stomach acid and _____ to form chyme.

3. Nutrients and fluids are absorbed into the _____ for use by the body's cells.

4. By the time the chyme reaches the rectum, it contains only waste material called _____.

Activity B *Place an "X" in front of the characteristics of feces that could be a sign of illness.*

1. _____ Feces are watery.

2. _____ Feces are black.

3. _____ Feces are soft and brown.

4. _____ Feces are formed with a distinct odor.

5. _____ Feces are dry and hard.

Activity C *Mark each statement as either "true" (T) or "false" (F). Correct the false statements.*

1. **T F** Drinking plenty of fluids makes bowel movements easier.

2. **T F** Regular exercise causes constipation.

3. **T F** Holding feces for too long can lead to diarrhea.

4. **T F** Warm fluids help to stimulate the bowels to empty.

5. **T F** Fiber adds bulk to the feces, causing them to hold fluid.

Activity D *Fill in the blanks using the words given in parentheses.*

(defecate, chyme, movement, anus)

1. In the stomach, the food is broken down and mixed with stomach acid and enzymes to form liquid _____.

2. The presence of feces in the rectum stimulates the urge to _____, and the feces leave the body through the _____. This process is called "having a bowel _____."

PROBLEMS WITH BOWEL ELIMINATION

Key Learning Points

- Problems with bowel elimination
- How to assist a person who is having problems with bowel elimination
- Observations that should be reported when assisting a person with bowel elimination
- The words *diarrhea, fecal impaction, flatus, flatulence,* and *fecal (bowel) incontinence*

Activity A *Place an "X" next to the statements that are true.*

1. _____ Frequent or excessive diarrhea can cause dehydration, especially in young or elderly people.

2. _____ Excess fiber in the diet can cause constipation.

3. _____ Laxatives are medications that help people with diarrhea.

4. _____ A person with a fecal impaction may complain of abdominal or rectal pain or of liquid feces "seeping" out of the anus.

5. _____ Flatus is a natural by-product of digestion.

6. _____ Incontinence briefs and bed protectors may be used to help manage fecal incontinence.

Activity B *Match the treatment, given in Column A, with its description, given in Column B.*

Column A

_____ 1. Laxative

_____ 2. Stool softener

_____ 3. Fiber supplement

_____ 4. Rectal suppository

_____ 5. Enema

_____ 6. Bowel training

Column B

a. Wax-like substance that dissolves at body temperature

b. Medication that chemically stimulates peristalsis

c. Solutions that are placed in the rectum

d. Medication that helps to keep fluid in the feces

e. Promotes regular, controlled bowel movements

f. Adds bulk to the feces, causing it to hold fluid

Activity C *Place an "X" next to observations that need to be reported to the nurse.*

1. _____ Presence of blood or mucus in the feces

2. _____ Soft, moist, formed stool

3. _____ Bleeding from the anus during or after bowel movement

4. _____ Liquid feces "seeping" from the anus

5. _____ Excessive flatus

Activity D *Match the words, given in Column A, with their definitions, given in Column B.*

Column A

_____ 1. Diarrhea

_____ 2. Fecal impaction

_____ 3. Flatus

_____ 4. Flatulence

_____ 5. Fecal incontinence

Column B

a. Inability to hold one's feces

b. Gas that is formed as part of the digestive process

c. Condition that occurs when constipation is not relieved

d. Passage of liquid, unformed feces

e. Presence of excessive amount of flatus in the intestines

OBTAINING A STOOL SPECIMEN

Key Learning Points

- How to collect a stool specimen
- The word *stool*

Activity A *Mark each statement as either "true" (T) or "false" (F). Correct the false statements.*

1. T   F   The specimen container should be labeled.

2. T   F   The specimen collection device should be lined with toilet paper before collection.

3. T   F   The person should not urinate into the specimen collection device.

4. T   F   A tongue depressor can be used to transfer the contents from the specimen collection device to the specimen container.

5. T   F   The uncovered specimen container containing the specimen should be placed into a transport bag.

ASSISTING WITH ENEMAS

Key Learning Points

- Conditions that may make use of an enema necessary
- Types of enemas
- How to administer an enema safely
- How to administer a soapsuds enema
- The word *enema*

Activity A *List three situations when a doctor may order an enema for a person.*

1. _____

2. _____

3. _____

Activity B *Match the type of enema, given in Column A, with its function, given in Column B.*

Column A

_____ **1.** Cleansing enema

_____ **2.** Oil retention enema

_____ **3.** Commercial enema

Column B

a. Administered to help relieve constipation and as a part of bowel training

b. Administered prior to diagnostic tests or surgery that involves the colon

c. Administered to help remove fecal impaction

Activity C *Fill in the blanks using the words given in parentheses.*

(fluid imbalance, pain, death, cramping)

1. If the enema solution is too cool, it may

cause abdominal _____

and _____.

2. If the enema solution is too hot, it may cause serious injury, possibly even

_____.

3. If too many enemas are given in one session, the person may develop a

_____ _____.

Activity D *Write down the correct order of the steps for giving a soapsuds enema in the boxes provided below.*

1. Position the person in the Sims' position.

2. Ask the person to exhale as the enema tubing is inserted.

3. Remove all air from the tubing.

4. Assist the person with expelling the enema and provide perineal care as necessary.

5. Mix warm water and castile soap in the enema bag.

6. Lubricate the tip of the enema tubing.

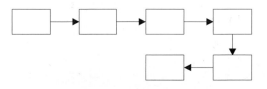

Activity E *Place an "X" next to the statements that are true about administering an enema.*

1. _____ An enema is a solution that is placed in the large intestine by way of the anus to remove feces from the rectum.

2. _____ The doctor may order an enema to relieve headaches.

3. _____ A nursing assistant only administers an enema if this task is within his or her scope of practice.

4. _____ An enema may be given to prepare the person for surgery or a diagnostic test.

5. _____ Contact with body fluids is likely when assisting with enemas.

ASSISTING WITH OSTOMY CARE

Key Learning Points

- Two common types of ostomies
- The emotional impact of having an ostomy
- Proper technique for providing routine ostomy care
- The word *ostomy*

Activity A *Match the words, given in Column A, with their definitions, given in Column B.*

Column A

_____ **1.** Ileostomy

_____ **2.** Colostomy

_____ **3.** Stoma

_____ **4.** Ostomy appliance

_____ **5.** Ostomy

Column B

a. The feces collect in this pouch, which is worn over the stoma

b. An alternate way of removing feces from the body

c. Ostomy in which the entire large intestine is removed

d. Ostomy in which only part of the large intestine is removed

e. An artificial opening made in the person's abdomen

Activity B *Fill in the blanks using the words given in parentheses.*

(stoma, ostomy, down, adhesive, skin)

1. The ostomy appliance is disconnected from the _____ belt.

2. Warm water or _____ solvent may be used to soften the adhesive to remove the ostomy appliance.

3. Cover the _____ with a gauze pad to absorb any drainage that may occur until the new appliance is in place.

4. Clean the skin around the stoma and apply the _____ barrier if needed.

5. Center the appliance over the stoma, making sure that the drain or the end of the bag is pointed _____.

Activity C *Identify the type of ostomy in the pictures below.*

1. _____

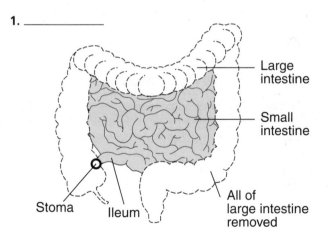

2. _____

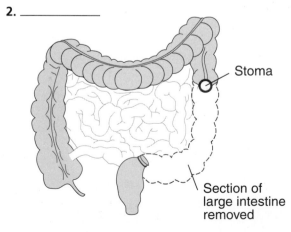

24

Assisting With Comfort

GENERAL COMFORT MEASURES

Key Learning Points

- The importance of rest and sleep
- Factors affecting a person's ability to rest and sleep in a health care setting
- Ways to promote rest and sleep
- Proper technique for giving a back massage

Activity A *Fill in the blanks using the words given in parentheses.*

1. _____ (Rest/Music) and sleep are basic physical needs.

2. When we are without _____ (food/pain) or distress, we are able to rest and relax.

3. Helping patients and residents to be as comfortable as possible is an important part of

   providing _____ (holistic/medical) care.

Activity B *Place an "X" next to the factors that can negatively affect a person's ability to rest and sleep in a health care setting.*

1. _____ The person may be in pain.

2. _____ There may be strange sounds or smells.

3. _____ Members of the health care team are talking loudly in the hall.

4. _____ The person is not used to having a roommate.

5. _____ The person may be worried about his family members who are at home.

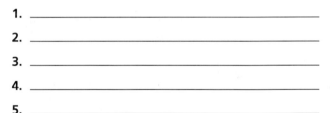 **Activity C** *Make a list of at least five things a nursing assistant can do to keep patients or residents as comfortable as possible.*

1. _____

2. _____

3. _____

4. _____

5. _____

Activity D *On the pictures below, draw the sequence of strokes for each phase of a back massage.*

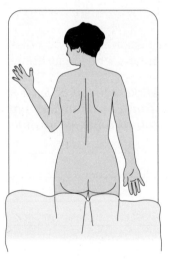

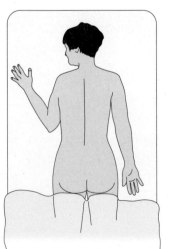

MANAGING PAIN

Key Learning Points

- Types of pain
- Factors affecting a person's response to pain
- Observations indicating signs of pain
- The importance of promptly reporting a person's pain to the nurse
- Medications used to control pain
- The nursing assistant's role in managing pain
- The words *acute pain* and *chronic pain*

Activity A *Mark each statement as either "true" (T) or "false" (F). Correct the false statements.*

1. **T F** Pain is the body's distress signal.

2. **T F** Acute pain increases as the body's tissues repair themselves and heal.

3. **T F** Chronic pain continues even after tissue healing has taken place.

4. **T F** Pain makes it difficult for a person to rest, relax, and sleep.

Activity B *Place an "X" next to the statements that are true.*

1. _____ A person's culture and upbringing can affect the way he responds to pain.

2. _____ A nursing assistant does not need to report a patient's or resident's pain to the nurse if the person does not complain about the pain.

3. _____ A person may try to be very courageous and ignore the pain.

4. _____ A person's past experience with pain can affect the way he responds to pain.

5. _____ A patient or resident can let a nursing assistant know that she is in pain using verbal or nonverbal communication.

Activity C *Select the single best answer for the following question.*

1. Which of the following could be a nonverbal sign of pain?
   a. A smile
   b. Vomiting
   c. Grimacing
   d. Constipation

Activity D *Think About It! Briefly answer the following question in the space provided.*

You are assisting Mrs. Meloney to the bathroom, when she complains of pain. Write down five questions you would ask Mrs. Meloney so that you will be able to provide the nurse with as much detail as possible about Mrs. Meloney's pain.

1. _____

2. _____

3. _____

4. _____

5. _____

Activity E *Mark each statement as either "true" (T) or "false" (F). Correct the false statements.*

1. **T F** It is important to promptly report a patient's or resident's pain to the nurse.

2. **T F** Pain can help a person to relax and sleep.

3. **T F** If left untreated the pain may subside on its own.

Activity F *List five things a nursing assistant can do to help a person in pain.*

1. _____

2. _____

3. _____

4. _____

5. _____

As a nursing assistant, one of the most important things you can do for your patients or residents is notice and report pain. If the pain is new, the nurse will need to find out what is causing the pain. Even if the pain is familiar and the cause of it is known, there may still be something the nurse can do to help make the person more comfortable.

Activity G *Fill in the blanks using the words given in parentheses.*

1. _____ (Acute/Chronic) pain may caused by conditions such as arthritis or cancer.

2. _____ (Acute/Chronic) pain occurs with an injury and lasts for a short period of time.

3. _____ (Acute/Chronic) pain continues even after tissue healing has taken place.

4. Acute pain _____ (increases/decreases) as the body's tissues repair themselves and heal.

HEAT AND COLD APPLICATIONS

Key Learning Points

- Use of heat and cold applications
- Safety concerns related to heat and cold applications
- Observations to be reported with regard to heat and cold applications
- Technique for giving a moist cold application
- Technique for giving a dry cold application
- Technique for giving a dry heat application

Activity A *Place an "X" next to each correct answer for the following questions.*

1. What are the uses of heat applications?

_____ **a.** Dilate the blood vessels

_____ **b.** Numb sensations and control bleeding

_____ **c.** Reduce fevers

_____ **d.** Relieve muscle spasms

2. What are the uses of cold applications?

_____ **a.** Reduce fevers

_____ **b.** Relieve pain and prevent swelling

_____ **c.** Promote circulation to speed healing

_____ **d.** Constrict blood vessels

Activity B *Think About It! Briefly answer the following question in the space provided.*

Some people are at very high risk for injury from the application of heat or cold. Briefly explain why heat and cold applications must be used with extreme caution in each of the residents described below.

1. Mr. Rider has dementia.

   _____

2. Mr. Jansen is of Scandinavian descent and has very fair skin.

   _____

3. Mrs. Klipinger has diabetes.

   _____

4. Mrs. Orwell is 93 years old.

   _____

Activity C *Place an "X" next to the observations that should be reported to the nurse when you are assisting a patient or a resident with heat and cold applications.*

1. _____ The skin is pale and does not return to its normal color quickly after a cold application is removed.

2. _____ Blisters appear after the application is removed.

3. _____ The person complains of pain or a burning sensation.

4. _____ The skin is bright red or very pale and does not return to its normal color quickly after a hot application is removed.

5. _____ The person does not feel the warmth of the heat application.

Activity D *Fill in the blanks using the words given in parentheses.*

1. A moist cold application requires the compress to be soaked in _____ (warm/ice) water.

2. The compress is placed on the required site of the person's body for _____ (5 to 10/ 15 to 20) minutes.

3. The skin beneath the compress is checked every _____ (5/10) minutes.

4. If the skin appears pale or _____, (red/blue) or if the person complains of numbness or burning sensation, discontinue treatment and notify the nurse.

Activity E *Write down the correct order of the steps for giving a dry cold application in the boxes provided below.*

1. The ice bag is wiped dry and wrapped in a towel.

2. The ice bag is checked for leaks.

3. The skin beneath the ice bag is checked every 10 minutes.

4. Excess air in the ice bag is squeezed out.

5. The ice bag is filled one-half to two-thirds full with crushed ice.

6. The ice bag is applied to the treatment site for 15 to 20 minutes.

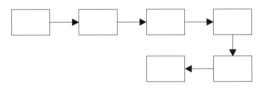

Activity F *Mark each statement as either "true" (T) or "false" (F). Correct the false statements.*

1. **T F** An aquamatic pad is used for giving a dry heat application.

2. **T F** The heating unit is filled with tap water.

3. **T F** The aquamatic pad is placed in a cover before applying it to the treatment area.

4. **T F** If the skin beneath the aquamatic pad appears red, swollen, or blistered, the treatment should be discontinued and the nurse notified.

5. **T F** You can use pins to secure the aquamatic pad to the treatment site.

25

Caring for People Who Are Dying

TERMINAL ILLNESS

Key Learning Points

- The stages of grief
- Communication techniques used to support a person during each stage of grief
- The role of hospice in the care of a terminally ill person
- The words *terminal illness, grief, hospice care, supportive care,* and *palliative care*

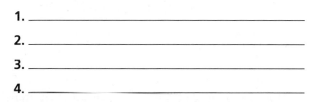 **Activity A** *Think About It! Briefly answer the following question in the space provided.*

List four diseases or conditions that can be considered terminal.

1. _____

2. _____

3. _____

4. _____

Activity B *Mark each statement as either "true" (T) or "false" (F). Correct the false statements.*

1. T F Focus on making the patient or resident comfortable and filling his last days with love and compassion.

2. T F Focus on the patient's or resident's physical as well as emotional and spiritual needs.

3. T F Avoid exploring your own feelings and emotions regarding death and dying.

4. T F A person who is dying may want to talk to you. Listen to whatever the person wants to say, and remember to be judgmental.

Activity C *Match the stages of grief, given in Column A, with their descriptions, given in Column B.*

Column A

_____ 1. Denial

_____ 2. Anger

_____ 3. Bargaining

_____ 4. Depression

_____ 5. Acceptance

_____ 6. Hope

Column B

a. The person wants to make a deal with someone he feels has control over his or her fate (e.g., God, a health care provider).

b. The person will bc sad and may have regrets about things he was not able to accomplish in his life.

c. The person refuses to accept the diagnosis or feels that a mistake has been made.

d. The person waits for new drugs that could act as a cure.

e. The person becomes moody, withdrawn, uncooperative, and hostile.

f. The person completes unfinished business and says his goodbyes.

Activity D Mark each statement as either "true" (T) or "false" (F). Correct the false statements.

1. **T F** As a nursing assistant, it is your duty to convince a terminally ill person that advances in medical technology can be of no help.

2. **T F** You must allow a terminally ill person to experience a feeling of hope, without being unrealistic.

3. **T F** When a family member of a terminally ill person directs her anger at you, you should take it personally.

4. **T F** You should try to ignore a terminally ill person who wants to talk to you about death.

5. **T F** Arranging for the assistance of clergy or other professionals experienced in grief counseling may be of great comfort to the person and the family.

Activity E Fill in the blanks using the words given in parentheses.

(supportive, emotional, grief, hospice, palliative)

1. Terminally ill people become eligible for

_____ care.

2. Hospice workers provide _____ care

and _____ care to keep the person as comfortable as possible as death approaches.

3. Hospice workers provide _____ support to both the terminally ill person and the family.

4. After the person dies, hospice workers continue to support the family by providing

_____ counseling.

Activity F Fill in the blanks using the words given in parentheses.

1. An illness or condition from which recovery

is not expected is called a _____ (casual/terminal) illness.

2. _____ (Acceptance/Grief) is mental anguish, specifically associated with loss.

3. _____ (Hospice/Quality) care is the term used for care provided by a health care organization for people who are dying, and for their families.

4. Treatments that will not prolong life, but will make a person more comfortable, such as oxygen therapy, nutritional supplementation, pain medication, and so forth, are called

_____ (supportive/palliative) care.

5. Care that focuses on relieving uncomfortable symptoms, not on curing the problem that is causing the symptoms, like chemotherapy or radiation to shrink a tumor, surgical procedures, and so forth, is called

_____ (supportive/palliative) care.

ADVANCE DIRECTIVES AND WILLS

Key Learning Points

- Ways that a person can specify wishes for end-of-life care in advance
- How a person can specify wishes for the management of his affairs after death
- The words *advance directive, living will, durable power of attorney for health care, do not resuscitate (DNR) order,* and *will*

Activity A *Fill in the blanks using the words given in parentheses.*

(durable power of attorney, DNR, life-sustaining, will, hospice, advance directive, living will)

1. A/An _____ _____ is a document that allows a person to make his wishes regarding health care known to family members and health care workers, in case the time comes when he is no longer able to make those wishes known himself.

2. A _____ _____ requests that death not be artificially postponed.

3. A _____ _____ _____ _____ for health care transfers the responsibility for handling a person's affairs and making medical decisions to a family member, friend, or other trusted individual, in the event that the person is no longer able to make these decisions on her own behalf.

4. A _____ (do not resuscitate) order written on a person's chart indicates that the person does not want the usual efforts to save her life to be made.

5. _____ agencies and facilities are organizations founded with the mission of offering the terminally ill person the best quality of life possible, and ensuring his comfort and dignity as death approaches.

6. A _____ is a legal statement that expresses a person's wishes for the management of her affairs after death.

7. _____ treatments, such as respiratory ventilation, cardiopulmonary resuscitation (CPR), or the placement of a feeding tube or intravenous (IV) line, are used to prolong life.

Activity B *Think About It! Briefly answer the following question in the space provided.*

You are caring for Mr. Thomas, a terminally ill patient. Mr. Thomas expresses a desire to make a will. What should you do?

_____

_____

_____

ATTITUDES TOWARD DEATH AND DYING

Key Learning Points

- Factors that can affect how a person views death
- Why it is important for health care workers to examine their own feelings about death
- The words *afterlife* and *reincarnation*

Activity A *Place an "X" next to the factors that can affect a person's attitude toward death.*

1. ____ Cultural beliefs
2. ____ Religious beliefs
3. ____ Previous experience with death
4. ____ Belief in reincarnation

Activity B *Think About It! Briefly answer the following question in the space provided.*

You have been caring for Mrs. Ford, who is now in the last stage of cancer. As you watch her family suffer and grieve, you feel helpless and emotionally drained. How would you cope with this situation?

_____

_____

_____

Activity C *Fill in the blanks using the words given in parentheses.*

(afterlife, reincarnation)

1. The idea that a person's soul will live again on earth in the form of an animal or human being yet to be born is called _____.

2. _____ is a state of being where the dead meet again with loved ones who have passed on before them.

CARE AND SUPPORT OF THE DYING PERSON AND THE FAMILY

Key Learning Points

- Physical changes that occur as death nears
- How to keep a dying person physically comfortable
- How to support a dying person emotionally
- Ways to help the family of a dying person

Activity A *Select the single best answer for each of the following questions.*

1. Which of the following is a physical sign of impending death?

    a. Increased pain

    b. Increased thirst

    c. Irregular, shallow breathing

    d. Increased urine output

2. Which of the following happens when circulation fails?

    a. The blood pressure rises.

    b. The pulse becomes rapid and weak.

    c. The skin feels warm.

    d. The body temperature falls.

3. Which of the following generally does NOT result from nervous system changes?

    a. Pain lessens

    b. Vision blurs

    c. Altered consciousness

    d. Diminished hearing

Activity B *Match the organ system, given in Column A, to the sign of impending death, given in Column B.*

Column A	Column B
_____ **1.** Circulatory	**a.** A person may experience nausea, vomiting, abdominal swelling, fecal impaction, or bowel incontinence.
_____ **2.** Respiratory	
_____ **3.** Digestive	
_____ **4.** Urinary	**b.** A person's blood pressure drops and the pulse becomes rapid and weak.

c. Output decreases.

d. A person may take very irregular, shallow breaths, in an alternating fast–slow pattern.

Activity C *Place a "P" next to the activities that a nursing assistant performs to meet a dying person's physical needs and an "E" next to activities that are performed to meet the person's emotional needs.*

1. _____ Providing frequent skin care

2. _____ Listening when the person wants to talk

3. _____ Providing frequent oral care

4. _____ Repositioning the person frequently

5. _____ Letting the person cry

6. _____ Asking a counselor to speak to the person about death

Activity D *Select the single best answer for each of the following questions.*

1. To make communication more effective, what kind of questions should you ask the dying person if she loses the ability to speak clearly?

    a. Open-ended questions

    b. "Fill in the blanks" questions

    c. "Yes or no" questions

    d. Multiple-choice questions

2. How would you respond if a family member expresses a wish to assist in providing physical care to the dying person?

    a. Encourage the family member by suggesting ways in which he can help.

    b. Assume that the family member will not be able to provide care to a dying person, as he has no formal training.

    c. Ask the family member to wait until you have finished caring for the dying person.

    d. Just say "I will have to ask the nurse about this."

3. Which of the following actions would let a person know that she is cared for and is not alone?

   a. Gently holding the person's hand or touching her shoulder when you are speaking to her

   b. Gently smoothing the person's hair after you have finished straightening the bed linens

   c. Sitting with the person quietly

   d. All of the above

Activity E *Place an "X" next to the statements that reflect behavior that may be an unconscious effort on the nursing assistant's part to avoid a person who is dying.*

1. _____ The nursing assistant does not check in on the dying person as often as she checks in on her other patients or residents.

2. _____ The nursing assistant provides only the necessary care and then leaves the person's room quickly, afraid that if she stays, the person will want to talk about death.

3. _____ The nursing assistant takes an interest in the person and allows the person to talk about death.

4. _____ The nursing assistant becomes attached to her patient or resident and feels concerned about the person's death.

5. _____ The nursing assistant acts overly cheerful when around the dying person.

Activity F *Fill in the blanks using the words given in parentheses.*

(help, basic needs, talk, competent, good communication, compassionate)

1. Ensure _____ _____ between the family members and the health care team.

2. Encourage family members to _____

   to the dying person and to _____ with the person's care.

3. Ensure that the family members' _____

   _____ are met.

4. Often, the most comforting thing to family members is in knowing that their loved one

   is receiving _____, _____ care.

POSTMORTEM CARE

Key Learning Points

- The nursing assistant's responsibilities following the death of a patient or resident
- The proper technique for providing postmortem care
- The words *postmortem care, rigor mortis, shroud,* and *autopsy*

Activity A *Mark each statement as either "true" (T) or "false" (F). Correct the false statements.*

1. T F   Postmortem care is the care of a person's body before the person's death.

2. T F   Postmortem care is necessary to prevent skin damage and discoloration.

3. T F   Rigor mortis is the stiffening of the muscles that usually develops within 2 to 4 hours of death.

4. T F   It is easy to position the body in proper alignment after rigor mortis occurs.

5. T F   An autopsy is an examination of the person's organs and tissues after the person has died.

6. T F   A shroud is a covering used to wrap the body of a person who has died.

Activity B *Select the single best answer for the following question.*

1. When preparing a person's body for the family to view after death, we do all of the following EXCEPT:

   a. Change the soiled bed linens

   b. Cover the person's face with a sheet

   c. Straighten up the room

   d. Collect the person's belongings

Activity C *Fill in the blanks using the words given in parentheses.*

1. The care of a person's body after the person's

   death is called _____ (hospice/postmortem) care.

2. A covering used to wrap the body of a person

   who has died is called a _____. (shroud/restraint)

3. An examination of a person's organs and tissues after the person has died, done to confirm or identify the cause of the person's

   death, is called an _____. (operation/autopsy)

4. The stiffening of the muscles that usually develops within 2 to 4 hours of death is

   called _____. (rigor mortis/paralysis)

Activity D *Write down the correct order of the steps for providing postmortem care in the boxes provided below.*

A. Wash the body and comb the hair.

B. Close the eyes by placing a moistened cotton ball on each eyelid.

C. Apply the shroud.

D. Dress the body in a clean gown and change the bed linens.

E. Remove any jewelry and place it in a plastic bag or an envelope for the family.

F. Draw the top linens over the person, forming a cuff at the shoulders.

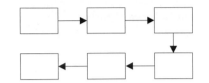

CHAPTER 26

Caring for People With Dementia

INTRODUCTION TO DEMENTIA

Key Learning Points

- The difference between dementia and delirium
- The words *dementia, activities of daily living (ADLs),* and *delirium*

Activity A *Mark each statement as either "true" (T) or "false" (F). Correct any false statements.*

1. **T F** Once the cause of dementia is identified and treated, the dementia will go away.

2. **T F** A person with dementia is likely to have problems with memory, especially short-term memory.

3. **T F** A person with dementia may act in socially inappropriate ways.

4. **T F** A person with dementia is able to make responsible decisions.

5. **T F** Dementia is a terminal illness.

Activity B *Fill in the blanks using the words given in parentheses.*

(dementia, delirium, activities of daily living)

1. Routine tasks of daily life, such as bathing, eating, and grooming are called

_____.

2. _____ is a temporary state of confusion that can be a symptom of an underlying disorder, such as an infection.

3. _____ is the permanent and progressive loss of the ability to think and remember, caused by damage to the brain tissue.

TYPES OF DEMENTIA

Key Learning Points

- The two most common types of dementia
- The stages of Alzheimer's disease

Activity A *Match the types of dementia, given in Column A, with their causes, given in Column B.*

Column A	Column B
_____ 1. Alzheimer's disease	a. Lack of blood flow to the brain resulting in tissue death
_____ 2. Vascular (multi-infarct) dementia	b. Plaques and tangles (abnormal protein deposits in brain)

Activity B *Think About It! Briefly answer the following question in the space provided.*

Barry's grandfather died of vascular (multi-infarct) dementia, and Barry is worried about his chances of developing the disease. List at least five risk factors for vascular (multi-infarct) dementia that Barry should be aware of.

_____

_____

_____

Activity C *A person with Alzheimer's disease passes through a number of stages. Identify whether the listed symptoms are mild, moderate, or advanced.*

1. The person needs help with dressing, although she can manage eating and toileting without help. The person is often disoriented to time and place and has trouble remembering the names of

   familiar people. _____

2. The person loses the ability to walk and sit independently. She is no longer able to speak, swallow, or smile. The person becomes totally incontinent of urine and

   feces. _____

3. The person begins to have trouble doing complex tasks, especially in social settings or at work (for example, calculating the tip

   on a restaurant check). _____

BEHAVIORS ASSOCIATED WITH DEMENTIA

Key Learning Points

- The behaviors that are common in people with dementia
- Strategies for managing difficult behaviors in people with dementia
- The word *validation therapy*

Activity A *Match the behaviors shown by people with dementia, given in Column A, with their descriptions, given in Column B.*

Column A

_____ 1. Wandering

_____ 2. Pacing

_____ 3. Repetition (perseveration)

_____ 4. Rummaging

_____ 5. Delusions

_____ 6. Hallucinations

_____ 7. Agitation

_____ 8. Catastrophic reactions

_____ 9. Sundowning

_____ 10. Inappropriate sexual behaviors

Column B

a. False beliefs

b. Searching through drawers or closets

c. Moving back and forth within a confined area

d. Doing the same thing over and over again

e. The person moves about without a specific destination in mind

f. Attempting to get into bed with another resident, or masturbating in a public area

g. Worsening of a person's behavioral symptoms in the late afternoon and evening, as the sun goes down

h. Becoming very upset and excited

i. Overreacting to something that would cause a healthy person minimal or no stress

j. Seeing, hearing, tasting, or smelling something that is not really there

Activity B *Mark each statement as either "true" (T) or "false" (F). Correct any false statements.*

1. T F A person with dementia may do the same thing over and over again. This is called pacing.

2. T F If one of your residents is delusional, try to correct the person.

3. T F Reality therapy stresses the importance of acknowledging the person's reality, rather than correcting the person.

Activity C *Match the behaviors seen in people with dementia, given in Column A, with actions that can be taken to help the person, given in Column B.*

Column A

_____ **1.** Wandering

_____ **2.** Pacing

_____ **3.** Repetition

_____ **4.** Rummaging

_____ **5.** Delusions

_____ **6.** Hallucinations

_____ **7.** Sundowning

_____ **8.** Inappropriate sexual behaviors

Column B

a. Use validation therapy

b. Ensure periods of quiet and rest during the day to reduce fatigue; turn on lights earlier in the evening

c. Reassure the person and then gently redirect the person's attention

d. Redirect the person's attention by introducing another activity

e. Allow the person to move around a safe area, such as an enclosed courtyard

f. Show the person a special drawer or a box filled with small personal items

g. Distract the person by offering to take her for a walk, or by getting her involved in an activity such as looking through a magazine

h. Move the person to a quieter area, offer a snack, or take the person to the bathroom

Activity D *Think About It! Briefly answer the following questions in the spaces provided.*

1. Mrs. Wyatt has dementia, and she shows many of the behaviors typical of people with dementia. In particular, she likes to wander and pace a lot. Lately, though, she has also been having more catastrophic reactions and showing more sundowning behavior as well. Why is it important to determine the cause of Mrs. Wyatt's behaviors, when everyone knows that these behaviors are "normal" for people who have dementia?

_____

_____

_____

2. Mr. Murphy has Alzheimer's disease. He insists that his son his coming to visit him today. Unfortunately, you know that his son died in a plane crash when he was 24, more than 20 years ago. How would you respond to Mr. Murphy?

_____

_____

_____

CARING FOR A PERSON WITH DEMENTIA

Key Learning Points

- Special considerations that the nursing assistant should keep in mind while helping a person with dementia with activities of daily living (ADLs)
- Special care measures that are taken to help maintain quality of life for a person with dementia
- The word *reminiscence therapy*

Activity A *Think About It! Briefly answer the following questions in the spaces provided.*

1. When you are helping a person with dementia with her activities of daily living (ADLs), there are things you can do to make the task at hand go more smoothly. List at least five of these things.

   _____
   _____
   _____

2. You work in a facility that cares exclusively for people with dementia. What special considerations would you have when you are assisting each of the following residents in the situations given?

   a. It is time for Mr. Rodriguez's tub bath.

   _____
   _____

   b. It is time for Mrs. Cheng to get dressed.

   _____
   _____

   c. Miss Myrtle is having lunch in the dining room.

   _____
   _____

   d. Mr. Rider needs to go to the bathroom.

   _____
   _____

3. List two types of therapy used to help meet the emotional needs of a person with dementia and give an example of each.

   _____
   _____
   _____
   _____

Activity B *Mark each statement as either "true" (T) or "false" (F). Correct any false statements.*

1. **T F** It is not necessary to assist a person with dementia with personal hygiene and grooming, since people with dementia cannot appreciate being clean and well groomed anyway.

2. **T F** When assisting a person with dementia with a task, it is important to use short words and short sentences.

3. **T F** A person with dementia cannot benefit from a kind word, a gentle touch, or a smile.

4. **T F** It is not important to help the person to maintain his independence because eventually he will be dependent on you for everything anyway.

5. **T F** People with dementia respond best to a calm, structured environment.

6. **T F** People with dementia can benefit from visual cues, such as a large "STOP" sign on the door or a large calendar in the person's room.

EFFECTS ON THE CAREGIVER

Key Learning Points

- How caring for a person with dementia can affect a nursing assistant
- Strategies that can help a nursing assistant to cope with the effects of caring for a person with dementia

Activity A *Mark each statement as either "true" (T) or "false" (F). Correct any false statements.*

1. **T F**   It is acceptable to physically punish a resident with dementia who has cursed at you, spit on you, slapped you, scratched you, pulled your hair, pinched you, or called you something offensive.

2. **T F**   Caring for a person with dementia is emotionally, but not physically, demanding.

3. **T F**   A person with dementia will be punished by a court of law if he causes any harm to the caregiver.

4. **T F**   When you become tired and frustrated, take time out, be good to yourself, and share your feelings with the nurse.

5. **T F**   If you get too angry with the person you should make sure the person is safe and walk away.

6. **T F**   If in your anger or frustration, you cause a patient or resident physical harm, you could lose your job.

Caring for People With Developmental Disabilities

INTRODUCTION TO DEVELOPMENTAL DISABILITIES

Key Learning Points

- Causes of developmental disabilities
- Eight common types of developmental disabilities
- The word *developmental disability*

Activity A *Fill in the blanks using the words given in parentheses.*

(acquired, oxygen, permanent, pregnancy, congenital)

1. A developmental disability is a _____ disability that interferes with the person's ability to achieve developmental milestones.

2. A developmental disability is _____ if the person was born with it.

3. A developmental disability is _____ if it occurred after the birth as a result of trauma or illness.

4. Consumption of alcohol, drugs, or other toxic substances during _____ can cause developmental disabilities.

5. Conditions that deprive a person of _____ can cause developmental disabilities.

Activity B *Mark each statement as either "true" (T) or "false" (F). Correct the false statements.*

1. **T F** A person with Down syndrome has certain characteristic physical features, such as eyelid folds that give the eyes an almond-shaped appearance; a large tongue in a small mouth; square hands with short, stubby fingers; a small, wide nose and small ears; short stature; and a wide, short neck.

2. **T F** A person with autism has extreme difficulty walking.

3. **T F** Varying degrees of mental retardation may accompany the physical disabilities associated with cerebral palsy.

4. **T F** Fetal alcohol syndrome is a combination of physical and mental problems that affect a child whose mother consumed alcohol during pregnancy.

5. **T F** People with autism may have above-average intelligence.

6. **T F** Some people with developmental disabilities are able to enter the workforce.

7. **T F** Spina bifida is a congenital defect of the spinal column.

8. T F Hydrocephalus results from a build-up of cerebrospinal fluid (CSF).

9. T F People who have fetal alcohol syndrome are usually moderately to severely mentally retarded and may have physical characteristics such as large, cupped ears; a slim build; wide-set, somewhat squinting eyes; and velvet-like skin.

EDUCATION AND PROTECTION OF RIGHTS

Key Learning Points

- Special education programs
- Laws and organizations

Activity A *Match the words, given in Column A, with their descriptions, given in Column B.*

Column A

_____ **1.** Self-care skills

_____ **2.** Life skills

_____ **3.** Social skills

_____ **4.** The Americans with Disabilities Act

_____ **5.** The Arc of the United States

Column B

a. Skills such as how to count money

b. Appropriate behavior and "limits" when interacting with other people

c. Ensures that people who have disabilities are treated the same as those without disabilities, by guaranteeing people with disabilities access to public education, employment, and public places such as parks, restaurants, and transportation

d. Promotes the rights of people with mental disabilities

e. Skills such as how to eat or dress independently

CARING FOR PEOPLE WITH DEVELOPMENTAL DISABILITIES

Key Learning Points

- Special considerations while helping a person with developmental disabilities with ADLs
- Methods used to help people with developmental disabilities maximize their abilities and become less dependent on others
- Observations that should be reported to the nurse when caring for a person with developmental disabilities

Activity A *List three considerations you should keep in mind while helping a person with developmental disabilities carry out activities of daily living (ADLs).*

1. _____

2. _____

3. _____

Activity B *Fill in the blanks using the words given in parentheses.*

(range-of-motion, assistive, physical)

1. Many people with developmental disabilities are able to manage their activities of daily living (ADLs) quite independently by using

_____ devices.

2. _____ rehabilitation may be used to maximize the person's independence and maintain levels of function.

3. _____ exercises are a form of physical rehabilitation.

Activity C *Place an "X" next to observations that need to be reported to the nurse when caring for a person with a developmental disability.*

1. _____ There is a change in the person's body temperature.

2. _____ The person's appetite does not show any signs of change.

3. _____ The person who is usually hyperactive now appears to be subdued.

4. _____ The person seems confused or disoriented.

5. _____ The person is always very aggressive.

6. _____ The person complains of pain or discomfort.

7. _____ The person shows signs of physical or mental abuse.

CHAPTER 28

Caring for People With Cancer

INTRODUCTION TO CANCER

Key Learning Points

- The difference between benign and malignant tumors
- Risk factors for cancer
- The words *tumor, benign, malignant,* and *metastasis*

Activity A *Fill in the blanks using the words given in parentheses.*

(malignant, benign, metastasis, kind, tumor, evil)

1. A _____ is an abnormal growth of tissue.

2. Tumors that are not cancerous are called

   _____.

3. Benign means _____.

4. Cancerous tumors are called _____.

5. Malignant means _____.

6. The process by which cancer cells spread from their original location in the body to a

   new location is called _____.

Activity B *Place an "X" next to the people who have risk factors for developing cancer.*

1. _____ A woman with a mother or sister who has breast cancer

2. _____ A person who smokes

3. _____ A person who exercises on a regular basis

4. _____ A person who spends a lot of time around people who smoke

5. _____ A person who works in a job that exposes him to radiation

6. _____ A person who lives in a damp, humid place

7. _____ A person who lives in a highly polluted town

8. _____ A person whose diet is high in fruit and vegetables

9. _____ A person whose diet is high in fat

DETECTING AND TREATING CANCER

Key Learning Points

- Early warning signs of cancer
- Importance of early detection of cancer
- Methods used to diagnose cancer
- Methods used to treat cancer
- The words *biopsy* and *prognosis*

Activity A *Fill in the blanks using the words given in parentheses.*

(cancers of the respiratory tract, skin cancer, cancers of the digestive system, bladder or kidney cancer, uterine cancer, oral cancer, colon cancer, breast cancer)

1. _____ Diarrhea or constipation or stool that has become smaller in diameter

2. _____ A sore that does not heal or small, scaly patches on the skin that bleed or do not heal

3. _____ A sore in the mouth that does not heal

4. _____ Unusual bleeding or discharge from the vagina

5. _____ Blood in the urine

6. _____ Thickening or lumps in and around the breast

7. _____ Indigestion, heartburn, or difficulty swallowing

8. _____ A cough that does not go away or a hoarse (rough) voice

Activity B *Think About It! Briefly answer the following question in the space provided.*

List the seven warning signs of cancer.

1. _____

2. _____

3. _____

4. _____

5. _____

6. _____

7. _____

Activity C *Fill in the blanks using the words given in parentheses.*

(endoscopic, screening tests, imaging studies, detection, biopsy)

1. Early _____ of cancer can lead to early treatment, which greatly improves a person's chances of surviving the disease.

2. _____ _____, such as x-rays, computed tomography (CT) scans, and magnetic resonance imaging scans, allow the doctor to see the tumor without actually entering the body.

3. _____ examinations involve using a lighted instrument to look inside the body and obtain tissue or fluids for analysis.

4. _____ can be performed by surgically removing all or part of the tumor, or by using a needle to obtain tissue or fluids for analysis.

5. Sometimes cancers are caught in their early stages through routine physical check-ups and _____ _____.

Activity D *Match the words, given in Column A, with their description, given in Column B.*

Column A

_____ 1. Surgery

_____ 2. Chemotherapy

_____ 3. Radiation

_____ 4. Prognosis

Column B

a. A doctor's estimation of the person's chances for recovery

b. Treatment for cancer using powerful x-ray beams that destroy cancer cells

c. Treatment for cancer involving removal of the tumor and surrounding tissues from the body

d. Treatment for cancer using medications that destroy cancer cells

CARING FOR A PERSON WITH CANCER

Key Learning Points

- Side effects of cancer treatment
- How to help a person who is experiencing side effects of cancer treatment feel more comfortable
- How cancer affects a person emotionally
- The words *alopecia* and *stomatitis*

Activity A *Given below are some side effects of treatments for cancer. Mark "C" if the side effect relates to chemotherapy, "R" if the side effect relates to radiation treatment, or "P" if the side effect relates to pain medication.*

1. _____ Nausea, vomiting, diarrhea, and loss of appetite

2. _____ Constipation

3. _____ Skin irritation

4. _____ Alopecia

5. _____ Stomatitis

Activity B *Write down the measures a nursing assistant can take to help minimize the following side effects.*

1. Pain

   _____

   _____

2. Nausea and vomiting

   _____

   _____

3. Skin irritation

   _____

   _____

4. Alopecia

   _____

   _____

5. Stomatitis

   _____

   _____

6. Fatigue

   _____

   _____

7. Increased risk for infection

   _____

   _____

Activity C *Think About It! Briefly answer the following questions in the spaces provided.*

1. List some of the fears a person who has been diagnosed with cancer might have.

   _____

   _____

   _____

2. How can you help the person cope with cancer emotionally?

   _____

   _____

   _____

CHAPTER 29

Caring for People With HIV/AIDS

INTRODUCTION TO HIV/AIDS

Key Learning Points

- How HIV infection affects the body
- Situations and behaviors that increase a person's risk of becoming infected with HIV
- The words *HIV-positive, acquired immunodeficiency syndrome (AIDS), homosexual,* and *heterosexual*

Activity A *Fill in the blanks using the words given in parentheses.*

(bloodborne, T cells, immune, immunodeficiency, HIV, infections)

1. Human immunodeficiency virus (HIV) is a

   _____ pathogen.

2. HIV invades the body's _____, special white blood cells that help to protect the body from infection.

3. As HIV takes over the body's _____ system, the infected person begins to have severe infections and rare cancers.

4. Most HIV-positive people eventually develop

   acquired _____ syndrome.

5. A person can be infected with _____ for many years before developing AIDS, or he may never develop AIDS.

6. AIDS is said to occur when the person's immune system is no longer able to fight off

   _____ and cancers.

Activity B *Place an "X" next to the factors that increase a person's risk of becoming infected with HIV.*

1. _____ Sharing needles

2. _____ Receiving tissue transplants

3. _____ Having unprotected sex

4. _____ Hugging an HIV-infected person

5. _____ Having an HIV-positive mother

6. _____ Transfusion of blood and blood products

Activity C *Match the words, given in Column A, with their definitions, given in Column B.*

Column A	Column B
_____ 1. HIV-positive	a. A person who is sexually attracted to members of the same sex
_____ 2. AIDS	
_____ 3. Homosexual	b. A person who is sexually attracted to members of the opposite sex
_____ 4. Heterosexual	

c. A disease caused by human immunodeficiency virus

d. The state of being infected with human immunodeficiency virus

ATTITUDES TOWARD PEOPLE WITH HIV/AIDS

Key Learning Points

- The rights of people with HIV/AIDS
- Measures to protect a person with HIV/AIDS from discrimination and poor treatment

Activity A *Think About It! Briefly answer the following question in the space provided.*

List three reasons a person with HIV/AIDS might experience discrimination.

1. _____

2. _____

3. _____

Activity B *Fill in the blanks using the words given in parentheses.*

(rights, AIDS, health, employment, discrimination)

1. A person with HIV/AIDS is at a risk for

_____.

2. Many states have laws designed specifically

to protect the _____ of people with HIV/AIDS.

3. Laws ensure the person's right to

_____, education, privacy, and health care.

4. In most states, people with _____ are protected under the Americans with Disabilities Act (ADA).

5. The nursing assistant protects the patient or resident from discrimination by keeping all

_____ information confidential.

CARING FOR A PERSON WITH HIV/AIDS

Key Learning Points

- Special considerations when providing physical care for a person with HIV/AIDS
- Emotional needs of a person with HIV/AIDS

Activity A *Match the physical problem of a person with HIV/AIDS, given in Column A, with its care measure, given in Column B.*

Column A

_____ 1. Painful sores in the mouth

_____ 2. Chronic diarrhea

_____ 3. Rashes and skin infections

_____ 4. Weakened immune system

_____ 5. Pain, weakness, and fatigue

Column B

a. Ask visitors with colds or contagious illnesses to delay visiting.

b. Use special cleansing agents and special bathing techniques.

c. Use a special numbing spray or mouthwash as ordered.

d. Assist the person with mild exercise combined with periods of rest to maintain muscle strength.

e. Serve nutritional supplements as ordered.

Activity B *Place an "X" next to the reasons people with HIV/AIDS may have emotional stress.*

1. _____ Many HIV-positive people are abandoned by friends and family members due to fear, shame, or disapproval.

2. _____ The person receives health care benefits because of the disease.

3. _____ The person may suffer from guilt, especially if risky behavior led to the infection.

CHAPTER 30

Caring for People Who Are Having Surgery

INTRODUCTION TO SURGERY

Key Learning Points

- Conditions that might make surgery necessary
- The words *peri-operative period, pre-operative phase, intra-operative phase,* and *postoperative phase*

Activity A *Place an "X" next to the statements that are true for surgery.*

1. _____ Surgery is used to diagnose and correct disorders.

2. _____ Surgery is used to repair injuries.

3. _____ Surgeries always have to be planned days in advance.

4. _____ Surgical procedures can be performed in a hospital or in an outpatient surgical center.

5. _____ After the surgery, the person is often discharged within a few hours to recover at home, in a subacute care facility, or in a long-term care facility.

Activity B *Fill in the blanks using the words given in parentheses.*

(peri-operative period, pre-operative phase, intra-operative phase, post-operative phase)

1. The phase before the surgery is actually performed, when the person is being prepared for the surgery, is called the

_____ _____.

2. During the _____ _____ the nursing assistant prepares a surgical bed for the person's arrival after the operation.

3. The _____ _____ involves a lot of care to prevent complications after surgery is actually performed.

4. The term used to describe all three phases of the surgical process as a whole is

_____ _____.

PRE-OPERATIVE CARE

Key Learning Points

- The role of the nursing assistant in helping a person to overcome his worries regarding surgery
- The role of the nursing assistant in preparing a person physically for surgery
- The purpose of a preoperative checklist
- The words *anesthesia* and *pre-operative teaching*

Activity A *Think About It! Briefly answer the following question in the spaces provided.*

Mr. Anderson is scheduled to have heart surgery tomorrow. List five things Mr. Anderson might be worried about. Then describe how a nursing assistant might help Mr. Anderson deal with these worries.

1. _____

2. _____

3. _____

4. _____

5. _____

Activity B *Mark each statement as either "true" (T) or "false" (F). Correct the false statements.*

1. **T   F**   A pre-operative checklist is used to confirm that all pre-operative tests and procedures have been completed and that informed consent has been obtained.

2. **T   F**   Anesthesia is loss of ability to feel pain due to an accident.

3. **T   F**   Pre-operative teaching is done by members of the health care team to prepare a person and his family for surgery.

4. **T   F**   A pre-operative checklist is completed before all other preparations have been made for surgery.

5. **T   F**   Doctors are often responsible for completing and recording many of the tasks on the pre-operative checklist.

INTRA-OPERATIVE CARE

Key Learning Points

- How to prepare the person's room for his or her arrival after surgery

Activity A *Fill in the blanks using the words given in parentheses.*

1. During the intra-operative phase, the

   nursing assistant prepares a _____ (surgical/open) bed for the person's arrival post-operation.

2. The bed is _____ (raised/lowered) to make it easier to transfer the person from the stretcher to the bed.

3. Furniture in the person's room is cleared to

   provide a pathway for the _____. (wheelchair/stretcher)

4. Supplemental _____ (oxygen/medication) should be kept ready in the person's room in preparation for post-operative care.

POST-OPERATIVE CARE

Key Learning Points

- Potential complications that may occur as a result of surgery and the measures taken to prevent them
- Observations that should be reported to the nurse when caring for a person who has just had surgery
- Proper technique for applying anti-embolism (TED) stockings
- The word *post-anesthesia care unit (PACU)*

Activity A *Place an "R" next to the statements that relate to post-operative respiratory complications and "C" next to the statements that relate to post-operative cardiovascular complications.*

1. _____ Drowsiness can make it difficult for the person to clear the lungs and the airways of fluid and mucus.

2. _____ The lungs may fill with fluid or collapse.

3. _____ Immobility can cause the body's circulation to slow down.

4. _____ Exchange of oxygen and carbon dioxide in the blood becomes difficult.

5. _____ Blood clots may move to lungs, heart, or brain.

6. _____ Sequential compression device (SCD), anti-embolism (TED) stockings, or leg exercises help to prevent clots.

7. _____ The person needs to be frequently repositioned and assisted with performing respiratory exercises.

Activity B *Think about it! Briefly answer the following question in the space provided.*

Post-operatively, what is the schedule for taking the person's vital signs? Why is it important to report a change in a surgical patients's vital signs immediately?

_____

_____

_____

_____

Activity C *Think About It! Briefly answer the following questions in the spaces provided.*

1. Look at the figure below. What respiratory exercise is the patient doing? What complications does this exercise help to prevent?

_____

_____

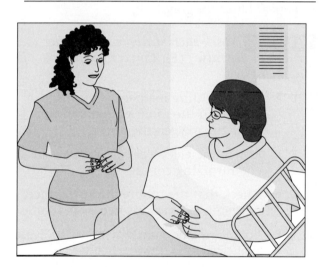

2. Look at the figure below. What respiratory exercise is the patient doing? What is the person supposed to do in this exercise?

_____

_____

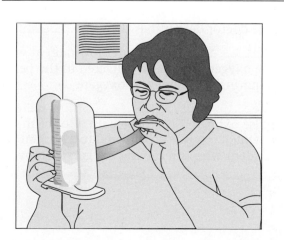

Activity D *Anti-embolism (TED) stockings apply pressure to the legs, helping to return blood to the heart and prevent cardiovascular complications of surgery, such as clot formation. Some of the steps for applying anti-embolism stockings are given below. Write down the correct order of the steps in the boxes provided below.*

1. Turn the stocking inside out down to the heel.

2. Grasp the top of the stocking and pull it up the person's leg.

3. Help the person into a comfortable position, straighten the bottom linens, and draw the top linens over the person. Ensure that the bed is lowered to its lowest position and that the wheels are locked.

4. Help the person into the supine position.

5. Slip the foot of the stocking over the person's toes, foot, and heel.

6. Make sure that the bed is positioned at a comfortable height and that the wheels are locked. Lower the side rail on the working side of the bed and keep the side rail on the opposite side of the bed up.

7. Fanfold the top linens to the foot of the bed and adjust the person's hospital gown or pajama bottoms as necessary to expose one leg at a time.

8. Check to make sure that the stocking is not twisted and that it fits snugly against the person's leg and over the heel and toe region.

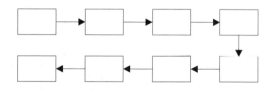

Activity E *Fill in the blanks using the words given in parentheses.*

(anesthesia, post-anesthesia, stable)

1. Immediately after surgery, the person is taken to the _____ care unit (PACU).

2. Once the person is awake, breathing normally, and has _____ vital signs, he or is moved from the PACU to a hospital room.

3. In the PACU, the person who has had surgery is closely monitored by the health care team to make sure that he or she is recovering without complications from the

surgery or the _____.

OXYGEN THERAPY

Key Learning Points

■ Conditions that might make oxygen therapy necessary
■ Three sources of oxygen for oxygen therapy
■ Two methods of delivering oxygen to the person
■ Observations that should be reported to the nurse when caring for a person who is receiving oxygen therapy
■ Safety guidelines that you should follow when caring for people receiving oxygen therapy
■ The word *flow meter*

Activity A *Match the words, given in Column A, with their descriptions, given in Column B.*

Column A

_____ **1.** Oxygen therapy

_____ **2.** Wall-mounted oxygen-delivery system

_____ **3.** Pressurized tank

_____ **4.** Oxygen concentrator

_____ **5.** Nasal cannula

_____ **6.** Face mask

Column B

a. A portable source of oxygen

b. Fits over the person's nose and mouth

c. A two-pronged device that is inserted into the person's nostrils

d. The oxygen is piped into the person's room from a central location

e. Administration of supplemental oxygen

f. Produces 100% oxygen by filtering the nitrogen out of the room air

Activity B *Place an "X" next to the observations that need to be reported to the nurse when caring for a person who is receiving oxygen therapy.*

1. _____ A reading above 85 percent on the pulse oximeter.

2. _____ The flow rate on the flow meter does not match the ordered flow rate.

3. _____ The pressure reading on the dial of a pressurized oxygen tank is low.

4. _____ The person breathes comfortably.

5. _____ There is an increase or decrease in respiratory rate.

6. _____ The person's lips, nailbeds, or face appear bluish or gray.

Activity C *Mark each statement as either "true" (T) or "false" (F). Correct the false statements.*

1. T F Avoid lighting matches or cigarette lighters in the room of the person receiving oxygen therapy.

2. T F Ensure the electrical equipment is in good working condition.

3. T F Check that the tubing through which oxygen is delivered is free of any kinks.

4. T F Bubbles in the humidity bottle indicate that oxygen is flowing freely.

5. T F The person is administered dry supplemental oxygen.

6. T F The nursing assistant can adjust the flow rate of oxygen.

Activity D *Fill in the blanks using the words in parentheses.*

1. The doctor determines the _____

_____ (temperature/flow rate) at which the oxygen should be delivered to the person requiring supplemental oxygen.

2. The _____ _____ (flow meter/ pulse oximeter) is a device used to set the rate at which oxygen is delivered to a patient or resident who is receiving oxygen therapy.

Introduction to the Language of Health Care

MEDICAL TERMINOLOGY

Key Learning Points

■ Roots, suffixes, prefixes, and combining vowels

Activity A *Break the following words into their roots, suffixes/prefixes, and combining vowels.*

1. Arthroscopy —————————

_____

2. Blepharoplasty —————————

_____

3. Cystitis —————————————

_____

4. Hepatomegaly ————————

_____

5. Nocturia ————————————

_____

6. Stomatitis ————————————

_____

7. Bradycardia ————————————

8. Hypogastric ————————————

_____

9. Pericarditis ————————————

_____

10. Intravascular ————————————

_____

11. Polydipsia ————————————

_____

12. Hyperemesis ————————————

_____

13. Leukocytopenia ————————————

_____

14. Electrocardiogram ————————————

_____

Activity B *Match the common roots, given in Column A, with their meanings, given in Column B.*

Column A	Column B
—— 1. Adip	a. Vessel
—— 2. Erythr	b. Eyelid
—— 3. Hepat	c. Fat
—— 4. Proct	d. Gallbladder
—— 5. Blephar	e. Red
	f. Bile, gall

—— 6. Cholecyst   g. Lower back

—— 7. Angi   h. Anus, rectum

—— 8. Lumb   i. Liver

—— 9. Chol

Activity C *Mark each statement as either "true" (T) or "false" (F). Correct the false statements.*

1. **T F** Retinopathy is a disease of the nose.

2. **T F** Hepatomegaly means enlargement of the liver.

3. **T F** Gastrectomy means removal of flatus from the stomach.

4. **T F** A glucometer is an instrument that is used to measure sugar (blood sugar.)

5. **T F** Scleroderma is hardening of the skin.

6. **T F** Hyperemesis means excessive vomiting.

Activity D *Fill in the blanks using the words given in parentheses.*

(prefixes, roots, suffixes, combining vowels)

1. _____ contain the essential, basic meaning of the word.

2. _____ and _____ are attached to the root to make the root more specific.

3. _____ _____ are often added in between the root and the suffix to make the new word easier to pronounce.

Activity E *Write the meaning of each of the following roots, suffixes, and prefixes.*

1. abdomin ————————————————

————————————————————————————

2. cephal ——————————————————

————————————————————————————

3. –centesis ————————————————

————————————————————————————

4. –gram ——————————————————

————————————————————————————

5. epi- ————————————————————

————————————————————————————

6. inter- —————————————————————

————————————————————————————————

7. peri- —————————————————————

————————————————————————————————

8. pre- —————————————————————

————————————————————————————————

9. tachy- ————————————————————

————————————————————————————————

10. –rrhaphy ————————————————————

————————————————————————————————

11. –scope ————————————————————

————————————————————————————————

12. –tome —————————————————————

————————————————————————————————

13. blephar ————————————————————

————————————————————————————————

14. encephal ————————————————————

————————————————————————————————

15. hemangi —————————————————————

————————————————————————————————

⬤ Make it a point to look up new words or abbreviations in a medical dictionary as soon as you hear or read them. Or, ask the nurse to explain the meaning of the word or the abbreviation to you. Before long, you will become very comfortable using and understanding the language of health care!

ANATOMICAL TERMS

Key Learning Points

■ Anatomical planes
■ Directional terms
■ The terms used to describe body cavities
■ The terms used to describe abdominal areas

Activity A *Mark each statement as either "true" (T) or "false" (F). Correct the false statements.*

1. **T F**   Health care professionals use specific terms to describe the location of one body part in relation to another.

2. **T F**   A person who is in normal anatomical position is standing upright and facing forward, with his feet close together.

3. **T F**   The sagittal plane is a horizontal plane that divides the body into upper and lower segments.

4. **T F**   Directional terms are used to describe the location of one body part in relation to the ground.

5. **T F**   Changing a person's body position changes the directional reference.

Activity B *Label the figure using the words given in parentheses.*

(frontal (coronal) plane, sagittal plane, transverse plane)

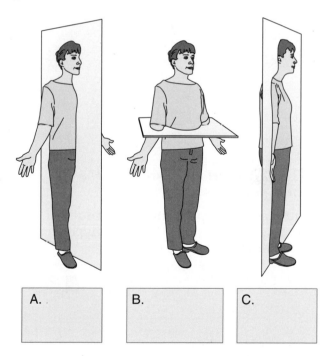

A.

B.

C.

Activity C *Fill in the blanks using the words given in parentheses.*

(anterior, superior, medial, inferior, posterior, lateral, distal, proximal)

1. The nose is ——————— to the eyes.

2. The ears are ——————— to the nose.

3. The eyes are ——————— to the breast.

4. The elbow is ——————— to the wrist.

5. The chest is ——————— to the throat.

6. The abdomen is ——————— to the buttocks.

7. The buttocks are ——————— to the abdomen.

8. The wrist is ——————— to the elbow.

Activity D *Mark each statement as either "true" (T) or "false" (F). Correct the false statements.*

1. **T F**   The dorsal cavity contains the brain and spinal cord.

2. **T F**   The ventral cavity is toward the back of the body.

3. **T F**   The ventral cavity is divided by the pleura into the thoracic (chest) cavity and the abdominal (belly) cavity.

4. **T F**   The thoracic cavity contains the lungs, the heart, and the large blood vessels.

5. **T F**   The lower abdominal cavity contains the stomach, liver, and pancreas.

6. **T F**   The upper abdominal cavity contains the urinary bladder, the rectum, and female reproductive organs.

Activity E *Label the figure using the words given in parentheses.*

(abdominal cavity, diaphragm, ventral cavity, dorsal cavity, thoracic cavity)

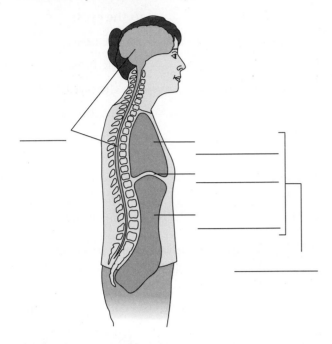

Activity F *Fill in the blanks using the words given in parentheses.*

(umbilical, hypogastric, epigastric, regions, iliac, quadrants)

1. _____ are typically used to describe general information, such as where a person is experiencing pain.

2. _____ are used when it is necessary to be very specific (for example, when describing where an incision is located).

3. The _____ and _____ regions are named for their relation to the stomach.

4. The _____ region is named for the belly button.

5. The _____ regions are also sometimes called the inguinal (groin) regions.

Activity G *Label the figure using the words given in parentheses.*

(left lower quadrant, left upper quadrant, right lower quadrant, right upper quadrant, umbilicus)

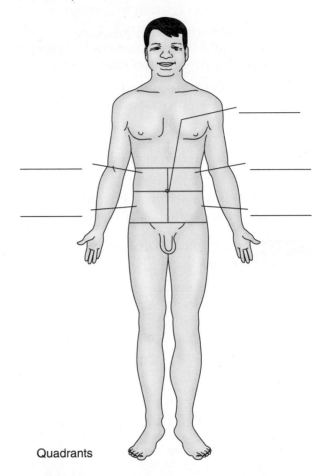

Quadrants

Activity H *Label the figure using the words given in parentheses.*

(right iliac, left hypochondriac, left lumbar, left iliac, epigastric, hypogastric, right hypochondriac, umbilical, right lumbar)

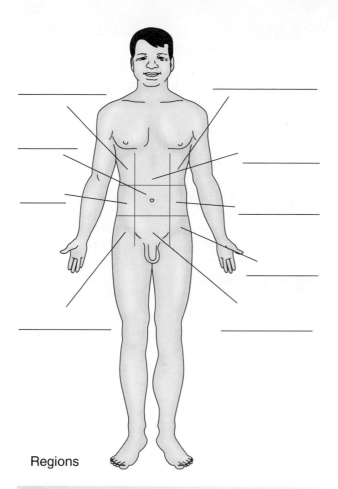

Regions

Understanding the terms and abbreviations that are unique to the health care profession is essential if you expect to be able to communicate effectively with other members of the health care team. Not knowing these terms and abbreviations will make it difficult for you to read and follow orders for patient or resident care. In addition, you will need to know these terms and abbreviations to accurately record and report.

ABBREVIATIONS

Key Learning Points

■ Abbreviations commonly used in health care

Activity A *Let's play* Jeopardy! *The category is "Medical Abbreviations." We'll give you the answer. You must pick the correct question from the four choices below.*

1. These are proteins made by the body to protect itself from foreign substances such as bacteria or viruses.
   a. What is Au?
   b. What is Ab?
   c. What is ac?
   d. What is Adm?

2. It is a hospital unit specially staffed and equipped to treat patients with serious cardiac problems.
   a. What is a CCU?
   b. What is a CHD?
   c. What is a CHF?
   d. What is a CBR?

3. It is a colorless, odorless gas, necessary for combustion and life.
   a. What is OB?
   b. What is OJ?
   c. What is O_2?
   d. What is O?

4. It is designed, equipped, and staffed to meet the needs of people who are recovering from anesthesia, regional blocks, and intravenous sedation.
   a. What is an OR?
   b. What is a PAR?
   c. What is a PM?
   d. What is a PT?

Activity B *Write the meaning for each of the following abbreviations.*

1. AIDS ————————————————

   ————————————————————

2. BKA ————————————————

   ————————————————————

3. CCU ————————————————

   ————————————————————

4. FBS ————————————————

   ————————————————————

5. HBV ————————————————

   ————————————————————

6. HIV ————————————————

————————————————

7. LPN ————————————————

————————————————

8. LVN ————————————————

9. NPO (npo) ——————————————

————————————————

10. qt ——————————————————

————————————————

11. R ——————————————————

————————————————

12. STD ————————————————

————————————————

13. Surg ——————————————

————————————————

14. WNL ——————————————

————————————————

15. wt ————————————————————

————————————————

Although abbreviations help save time and space when recording, it is very important to use only abbreviations that are approved for use in your facility. Otherwise, other members of the health care team may be confused by the meaning. If you are unsure of the meaning of an abbreviation, either look the abbreviation up, or ask the nurse to explain it.

CHAPTER 10 PROCEDURE CHECKLISTS

PROCEDURE 10-1
Handwashing

	S	U	COMMENTS
1. Gather needed supplies, if not present at the handwashing area: soap or the cleansing agent specified by your facility, hand lotion (optional), paper towels, a nailbrush (optional), an orange stick (optional).	☐	☐	_____
2. Stand away from the sink, so that your uniform does not touch the sink. Push your sleeves up your arms 4 to 5 inches; if you are wearing a watch, push it up too.	☐	☐	_____
3. Use a clean paper towel to turn on the faucet, adjusting the water temperature until it is warm. Dispose of the paper towel in a facility-approved waste container.	☐	☐	_____
4. Wet your hands, keeping your fingers pointed down. This will cause the water to run off your fingertips and into the sink. Do not allow water to run up your forearms.	☐	☐	_____
5. Press the hand pump or step on the foot pedal to dispense the cleaning agent into one cupped hand.	☐	☐	_____
6. Lather well, keeping your fingers pointed down at all times. Make sure the lather extends at least 1 inch past your wrists.	☐	☐	_____
7. Rub your hands together in a circular motion, washing the palms and backs of your hands. Interlace your fingers to clean the spaces between your fingers. Continue for at least 15 seconds.	☐	☐	_____
8. Rub the fingernails of one hand against the palm of the opposite hand to force soap underneath the tips of the fingernails, or clean underneath the tips of the fingernails with the blunt edge of an orange stick or a nailbrush.	☐	☐	_____
9. Rinse your hands, keeping your fingers pointed down at all times.	☐	☐	_____
10. Dry your hands thoroughly with a clean paper towel. Dispose of the paper towel in a facility-approved waste container, being careful not to touch the container.	☐	☐	_____
11. With a new paper towel, turn off the faucet. Carefully dispose of the paper towel.	☐	☐	_____

12. As you leave the handwashing area, if there is a doorknob, open the door by covering the doorknob with a clean paper towel. If there is no doorknob, push the door open with your hip and shoulder to avoid contaminating your clean hands.

☐ ☐ _____

13. After leaving the handwashing area, apply a small amount of hand lotion to keep your skin supple and moist.

☐ ☐ _____

PROCEDURE 10-2
Removing Gloves

	S	U	COMMENTS

1. With one gloved hand, grasp the other glove at the palm and pull the glove off your hand. Keep the glove you have removed in your gloved hand. (Think, "glove to glove.")   ☐ ☐ _____

2. Slip two fingers from the ungloved hand underneath the cuff of the remaining glove, at the wrist. Remove that glove from your hand, turning it inside-out as you pull it off. (Think, "skin to skin.")   ☐ ☐ _____

3. Dispose of the soiled gloves in a facility-approved waste container.   ☐ ☐ _____

4. Wash your hands.   ☐ ☐ _____

PROCEDURE 10-3
Putting on a Gown

	S	U	COMMENTS
1. Gather needed supplies: a gown, gloves.	☐	☐	_____
2. Remove your watch and place it on a clean paper towel or in your pocket. (If you are wearing jewelry, remove that as well.) Roll up the sleeves of your uniform so that they are about 4–5 inches above your wrists.	☐	☐	_____
3. Wash your hands.	☐	☐	_____
4. Put on the gown by slipping your arms into the sleeves.	☐	☐	_____
5. Secure the gown around your neck by tying the ties in a simple bow or by fastening the Velcro™ strips.	☐	☐	_____
6. Reach behind yourself and overlap the edges of the gown so that your uniform is completely covered. Secure the gown at your waist by tying the ties in a simple bow or by fastening the Velcro™ strips.	☐	☐	_____
7. Put on the gloves. The cuffs of the gloves should extend over the cuffs of the gown.	☐	☐	_____

PROCEDURE 10-4
Removing a Gown

	S	U	COMMENTS
1. Untie the waist ties (or undo the Velcro™ strips at the waist).	☐	☐	_____
2. Remove and dispose of your gloves as described in Procedure 10-2.	☐	☐	_____
3. Untie the neck ties (or undo the Velcro™ strips at the neck). Be careful not to touch your neck or the outside of the gown.	☐	☐	_____
4. Grasping the gown at the neck ties, loosen it at the neck.	☐	☐	_____
5. Slip the fingers of your dominant hand under the cuff of the gown on the opposite sleeve, and pull the sleeve over your hand. Be careful not to touch the outside of the gown with either hand.	☐	☐	_____
6. Use your gown-covered hand to pull the sleeve over your other hand, and then pull the gown off both arms.	☐	☐	_____
7. Holding the gown away from your body, roll it downward, turning it inside out as you go. Take care to touch only the noncontaminated side of the gown.	☐	☐	_____
8. After the gown is rolled up, contaminated side inward, dispose of it in a facility-approved container.	☐	☐	_____
9. Wash your hands.			

PROCEDURE 10-5
Putting on and Removing a Mask

Putting on a Mask

	S	U	COMMENTS
1. Gather needed supplies: a mask.	☐	☐	_____
2. Wash your hands.	☐	☐	_____
3. Place the mask over your nose and mouth, being careful not to touch your face with your hands.	☐	☐	_____
4. Tie the top strings of the mask securely behind your head.	☐	☐	_____
5. Tie the bottom strings of the mask securely behind your neck. Make sure that the mask fits snugly around your face. You want to breathe through the mask, not around it.	☐	☐	_____

Removing a Mask

	S	U	COMMENTS
1. Wash your hands. (You do not want to touch your face with dirty hands.)	☐	☐	_____
2. Untie the bottom strings first, and then untie the top strings.	☐	☐	_____
3. Remove the mask by holding the top strings. Dispose of the mask, holding it by its ties only, in the facility-approved container located inside the patient's or resident's room.	☐	☐	_____
4. Wash your hands.	☐	☐	_____

PROCEDURE 10-6
Double-Bagging (Two Assistants)

	S	U	COMMENTS

1. The nursing assistant inside the person's room places the contaminated items into an isolation bag (usually a color-coded plastic bag) and secures the bag with a tie. ☐ ☐ _____

2. Another nursing assistant, referred to as the "clean" nursing assistant, stands outside of the person's room, holding a plastic bag cuffed over her hands. The cuff at the top of the bag protects the "clean" nursing assistant's hands. ☐ ☐ _____

3. The nursing assistant inside the isolation unit deposits the bag of contaminated items into the bag held by the "clean" nursing assistant. ☐ ☐ _____

4. The "clean" nursing assistant secures the top of the plastic bag tightly and disposes of the double-bagged items according to facility policy. ☐ ☐ _____

CHAPTER 12 PROCEDURE CHECKLISTS

PROCEDURE 12-1
Applying a Vest Restraint

Getting Ready	S	U	COMMENTS
1. Complete the "Getting Ready" steps.	☐	☐	_____

Procedure

	S	U	COMMENTS
2. Get help from a nurse or another nursing assistant, if necessary.	☐	☐	_____
3. Assist the person to a sitting position by locking arms with her.	☐	☐	_____
4. Support the person's back and shoulders with one arm while slipping the person's arms through the armholes of the vest using your other hand. Apply the restraint according to the manufacturer's instructions. The vest should cross in the front, across the person's chest.	☐	☐	_____
5. Make sure there are no wrinkles across the front or back of the restraint.	☐	☐	_____
6. Bring the ties through the slots.	☐	☐	_____
7. Help the person to lie or sit down.	☐	☐	_____
8. Make sure the person is comfortable and in good body alignment.	☐	☐	_____
9. If the person is in a chair, thread the straps *between* the seat and the armrest or *between* the back of the seat and the back of the chair, according to the manufacturer's directions. If the person is in bed, attach the straps to the bed frame, never the side rails. Always use the quick-release knot approved by your facility.	☐	☐	_____
10. Make sure the restraint is not too tight. You should be able to slide a flat hand between the restraint and the person. Adjust the straps if necessary.	☐	☐	_____

Finishing Up

	S	U	COMMENTS
11. Complete the "Finishing Up" steps.	☐	☐	_____
12. Check on the restrained person every 15 minutes.	☐	☐	_____
13. Release the restraint every 2 hours and:			
a. Reposition the person.	☐	☐	_____
b. Meet the person's needs for food, fluids, and elimination.	☐	☐	_____
c. Give skin care and perform range-of-motion exercises.	☐	☐	_____

14. Reapply the restraint. □ □ _____

15. Report and record the procedure, noting the type □ □ _____
    of restraint used, the time the restraint was
    applied, and the person's response to the restraint.
    Include any other relevant observations and sign
    the chart. Be sure to include your title as well as
    your name.

PROCEDURE 12-2
Applying Wrist or Ankle Restraints

Getting Ready	S	U	COMMENTS
1. Complete the "Getting Ready" steps.	☐	☐	_____

Procedure

	S	U	COMMENTS
2. Get help from a nurse or another nursing assistant, if necessary.	☐	☐	_____
3. Apply the wrist or ankle restraint following the manufacturer's instructions. Place the soft part of the restraint against the skin.	☐	☐	_____
4. Secure the restraint so that it is snug, but not tight. You should be able to slide two fingers under the restraint.	☐	☐	_____
5. Attach the straps to the bed frame. Always use the quick-release knot approved by your facility.	☐	☐	_____
6. If applying more than one restraint, repeat steps 3 through 5.	☐	☐	_____

Finishing Up

	S	U	COMMENTS
7. Complete the "Finishing Up" steps.	☐	☐	_____
8. Check on the restrained person every 15 minutes.	☐	☐	_____
9. Release the restraint every 2 hours and:			
a. Reposition the person.	☐	☐	_____
b. Meet the person's needs for food, fluids, and elimination.	☐	☐	_____
c. Give skin care and perform range-of-motion exercises.	☐	☐	_____
10. Reapply the restraint.	☐	☐	_____
11. Report and record the procedure, noting the type of restraint used, the time the restraint was applied, and the person's response to the restraint. Include any other relevant observations and sign the chart. Be sure to include your title as well as your name.	☐	☐	_____

PROCEDURE 12-3
Applying Lap or Waist (Belt) Restraints

Getting Ready	S	U	COMMENTS
1. Complete the "Getting Ready" steps.	☐	☐	_____

Procedure

	S	U	COMMENTS
2. Get help from a nurse or another nursing assistant, if necessary.	☐	☐	_____
3. If the person is in a chair, assist him to a proper sitting position, making sure that the person's hips are as far back against the back of the chair as possible. (If the person is in a wheelchair, make sure the brakes are locked first, and position the footrests to support the person's feet.)	☐	☐	_____
4. Wrap the restraint around the person's abdomen, crossing the straps behind the person's back.	☐	☐	_____
5. Bring the ties through the loops at the sides of the restraint, according to the manufacturer's directions.	☐	☐	_____
6. Make sure the person is comfortable and in good body alignment.	☐	☐	_____
7. Thread the straps between the chair arm and the chair back before securing the straps out of the person's reach, at the back of the chair. Always use the quick-release knot approved by your facility.	☐	☐	_____
8. Secure the restraint, making sure it is not too tight. You should be able to slide a flat hand between the restraint and the person.	☐	☐	_____

Finishing Up

	S	U	COMMENTS
9. Complete the "Finishing Up" steps.	☐	☐	_____
10. Check on the restrained person every 15 minutes.	☐	☐	_____
11. Release the restraint every 2 hours and:			
a. Reposition the person.	☐	☐	_____
b. Meet the person's needs for food, fluids, and elimination.	☐	☐	_____
c. Give skin care and perform range-of-motion exercises.	☐	☐	_____
12. Reapply the restraint.	☐	☐	_____
13. Report and record the procedure, noting the type of restraint used, the time the restraint was applied, and the person's response to the restraint. Include any other relevant observations and sign the chart. Be sure to include your title as well as your name.	☐	☐	_____

CHAPTER 13 PROCEDURE CHECKLISTS

PROCEDURE 13-1
Relieving an Obstructed Airway in Conscious Adults and Children Older Than 1 Year

	S	U	COMMENTS

1. Check the person's ability to breathe and speak by tapping her on the shoulder and saying, "Are you okay? Can you talk? I can help you." A person who cannot breathe or speak needs immediate help. ☐ ☐ _____

2. If the person starts to cough, wait and see whether the coughing will dislodge the object. If the person's cough is weak and ineffective, or if the person is in obvious distress, continue with step 3. ☐ ☐ _____

3. Stay with the person and call for help. Have the person who is helping you activate the facility's emergency response system. ☐ ☐ _____

4. Stand behind the person with the obstructed airway and wrap your arms around her waist. ☐ ☐ _____

5. Make a fist with one hand and place the thumb of the fist against the person's abdomen, just above the navel and below the sternum (breastbone). Grasp your fist with the other hand. ☐ ☐ _____

6. Being careful not to put pressure on the person's ribs or sternum with your forearms, press your fist inward and pull upward, using quick thrusting motions, until the object is expelled, the person begins to cough forcefully, or the person loses consciousness. (In a child, less force is applied to the abdomen to avoid injuring the child's ribs, sternum (breastbone), and internal organs.)

    a. If the object is expelled, stay with the person, and follow the nurse's directions. ☐ ☐ _____

    b. If the person begins to cough, wait and see whether the coughing results in expulsion of the object. If it does not, continue giving abdominal thrusts. ☐ ☐ _____

    c. If the person loses consciousness, lower the person to the floor and begin Procedure 13-2, beginning with step 3. ☐ ☐ _____

7. The person should be evaluated by a doctor following the choking incident. ☐ ☐ _____

PROCEDURE 13-2

Relieving an Obstructed Airway in Unconscious Adults and Children Older Than 1 Year

	S	U	COMMENTS

1. Check the person's state of consciousness by gently shaking or tapping her. An unresponsive person needs immediate help.

2. Stay with the person and call for help. Have the person who is helping you activate the facility's emergency response system.

3. **Head tilt/chin lift maneuver.** Position the person on her back on a hard, flat surface. Open the person's airway by tilting the head back and lifting the chin. Look, feel, and listen for signs of breathing.

4. **Rescue breathing.** If the person is not breathing, keep her head tilted back and the chin lifted. Blow two slow breaths into the person's mouth through a ventilation barrier device, removing your mouth from the device and inhaling between each breath. If the air does not go in, repeat the head tilt/chin lift maneuver and attempt rescue breathing once again.

5. **Object check.** If no air enters the person's lungs after the second attempt, perform an object check. Kneel beside the person's head and open the airway using the head tilt/chin lift maneuver. Look for the object. If you see the object, remove it. If you cannot see the object, continue to step 6.

6. Repeat the head tilt/chin lift maneuver. Blow two slow breaths into the person's mouth through a ventilation barrier device, removing your mouth from the device and inhaling between each breath. If the air does not go in, repeat the head lift/chin tilt maneuver and attempt rescue breathing once again.

7. **Chest compressions.** If no air enters the person's lungs after the second attempt, begin chest compressions. To give chest compressions to an unconscious person:

   a. Kneel beside the person.

   b. Place the heel of your hand closest to the person's head on his sternum (breastbone) and place your other hand on top and interlock your fingers.

   c. Position your body forward so that your shoulders are over the center of the person's chest and your arms are straight. You will want to compress straight down and up. Do not rock back and forth.

   d. Compress the chest 1½ to 2 inches on an adult (1 to 1½ inches on a child) quickly at a rate of 100 compressions per minute for 30 compressions.

8. Perform an object check. ☐ ☐ _____

9. Repeat the head tilt/chin lift maneuver. Blow two breaths into the person's mouth through a ventilation barrier device, removing your mouth from the device and inhaling between each breath. If the air does not go in, repeat the head tilt/chin lift maneuver and attempt rescue breathing once again. ☐ ☐ _____

PROCEDURE 13-3

Relieving an Obstructed Airway in an Obese or Pregnant Person

	S	U	COMMENTS

1. Stand behind the person and place your arms under the person's armpits and around her chest. ☐ ☐ _____

2. Make a fist with one hand and place the thumb of the fist against the center of the person's sternum. Be sure that your thumb is centered on the sternum, not on the lower tip of the sternum (the xiphoid process) and not on the ribs. ☐ ☐ _____

3. Give up to five quick chest thrusts by grasping your fist with your other hand and pressing inward five times. Each thrust should compress the chest 1½ to 2 inches. ☐ ☐ _____

4. Continue to give chest thrusts until the object is expelled, the person begins to cough forcefully, or the person loses consciousness.

   a. If the object is expelled, stay with the person, and follow the nurse's directions. ☐ ☐ _____

   b. If the person begins to cough, wait and see whether the coughing results in expulsion of the object. If it does not, continue giving chest thrusts in groups of five. ☐ ☐ _____

   c. If the person loses consciousness, lower the person to the floor and follow the steps to Procedure 13-2. ☐ ☐ _____

5. The person should be evaluated by a doctor following the choking incident. ☐ ☐ _____

6. Record your observations and actions according to facility policy. ☐ ☐ _____

CHAPTER 14 PROCEDURE CHECKLISTS

PROCEDURE 14-1

Moving a Person to the Side of the Bed (One Assistant)

Getting Ready

	S	U	COMMENTS
1. Complete the "Getting Ready" steps.	☐	☐	_____

Procedure

	S	U	COMMENTS
2. Make sure that the bed is positioned at a comfortable working height (to promote good body mechanics) and that the wheels are locked.	☐	☐	_____
3. Place the pillow at the head of the bed, on its edge against the headboard. This gets the pillow out of the way.	☐	☐	_____
4. If the side rails are in use, lower the side rail on the working side of the bed. The side rail on the opposite side of the bed should remain up. Lower the head of the bed so that the bed is flat (as tolerated). Fanfold the top linens to the foot of the bed.	☐	☐	_____
5. Stand at the side of the bed with your feet spread about 12 inches apart and with your knees slightly bent to protect your back.	☐	☐	_____
6. Gently slide your hands under the person's head and shoulders and move the person's upper body toward you.	☐	☐	_____
7. Gently slide your hands under the person's torso and move the person's torso toward you.	☐	☐	_____
8. Gently slide your hands under the person's hips and legs and move the person's lower body toward you.	☐	☐	_____
9. Now, position the person as planned (e.g., in the prone or lateral position).	☐	☐	_____
10. Reposition the pillow under the person's head and straighten the bottom linens. Draw the top linens over the person. Raise the head of the bed as the person requests.	☐	☐	_____
11. Make sure that the bed is lowered to its lowest position and that the wheels are locked. If the side rails are in use, return them to the raised position.	☐	☐	_____

Finishing Up

	S	U	COMMENTS
12. Complete the "Finishing Up" steps.	☐	☐	_____

PROCEDURE 14-2

Moving a Person to the Side of the Bed (Two Assistants)

Getting Ready	S	U	COMMENTS
1. Complete the "Getting Ready" steps.	☐	☐	

Procedure

	S	U	COMMENTS
2. Make sure that the bed is positioned at a comfortable working height (to promote good body mechanics) and that the wheels are locked.	☐	☐	
3. Place the pillow at the head of the bed, on its edge against the headboard. This gets the pillow out of the way.	☐	☐	
4. If the side rails are in use, lower the side rails. Lower the head of the bed so that the bed is flat (as tolerated). Fanfold the top linens to the foot of the bed.	☐	☐	
5. If the lift sheet is already on the bed, make sure that it is positioned so that it is under the person's shoulders and hips. (If a lift sheet is not already on the bed, position one under the person's shoulders and hips.)	☐	☐	
6. Stand at the side of the bed, opposite your co-worker, with your feet spread about 12 inches apart and with your knees slightly bent to protect your back.	☐	☐	
7. Grasp the edge of the lift sheet and roll it over as close to the person's body as possible. This will provide for a better grip. (Your co-worker does the same.)	☐	☐	
8. Grasp the rolled edge of the lift sheet with both hands, palms and fingers facing down. One hand should be level with the person's shoulders and the other should be level with his or her hips.	☐	☐	
9. On the count of "three," slowly and carefully lift up on the lift sheet in unison and move the person to the side of the bed.	☐	☐	
10. Now, position the person as planned (e.g., in the prone or lateral position).	☐	☐	
11. Reposition the pillow under the person's head and straighten the bottom linens. Draw the top linens over the person.	☐	☐	
12. Make sure that the bed is lowered to its lowest position and that the wheels are locked. If the side rails are in use, return them to the raised position.	☐	☐	

Finishing Up

	S	U	COMMENTS
13. Complete the "Finishing Up" steps.	☐	☐	

PROCEDURE 14-3
Moving a Person up in Bed (One Assistant)

Getting Ready	S	U	COMMENTS
1. Complete the "Getting Ready" steps.	☐	☐	_____

Procedure

	S	U	COMMENTS
2. Make sure that the bed is positioned at a comfortable working height (to promote good body mechanics) and that the wheels are locked.	☐	☐	_____
3. If the side rails are in use, lower the side rail on the working side of the bed. The side rail on the opposite side of the bed should remain up. Fanfold the top linens to the foot of the bed.	☐	☐	_____
4. Place the pillow at the head of the bed, on its edge against the headboard. This gets the pillow out of the way. It also pads the headboard in case you move the person up a little too much or too fast!	☐	☐	_____
5. Method "A":			
a. Face the head of the bed. Position your outside foot (i.e., the foot that is farthest away from the edge of the bed) 12 inches in front of the other foot and bend your knees slightly to protect your back.	☐	☐	_____
b. Place your arm that is nearest the head of the bed under the person's head and shoulders. Lock your other arm with the person's arm that is closest to you.	☐	☐	_____
c. Have the person bend her knees.	☐	☐	_____
d. Tell the person that on the count of "three," she is to lift her buttocks and press her heels into the mattress as you lift her shoulders. On the count of "three," help the person to move smoothly toward the head of the bed.	☐	☐	
6. Method "B":			
a. Have the person grasp the head of the bed or a trapeze, if there is one.	☐	☐	_____
b. Face the head of the bed. Position your outside foot (i.e., the foot that is farthest away from the edge of the bed) 12 inches in front of the other foot and bend your knees slightly to protect your back.	☐	☐	_____
c. Place your hands under the person's back and buttocks.	☐	☐	_____
d. Have the person bend his knees.	☐	☐	_____
e. Tell the person that on the count of "three," he is to lift his buttocks and press his heels into the mattress. On the count of "three," help the person to move smoothly toward the head of the bed.	☐	☐	_____

7. Reposition the pillow under the person's head and straighten the bottom linens. Draw the top linens over the person. Raise the head of the bed as the person requests. ☐ ☐ _____

8. Make sure that the bed is lowered to its lowest position and that the wheels are locked. If the side rails are in use, return them to the raised position. ☐ ☐ _____

Finishing Up

9. Complete the "Finishing Up" steps. ☐ ☐ _____

PROCEDURE 14-4
Moving a Person up in Bed (Two Assistants)

	S	U	COMMENTS

Getting Ready

1. Complete the "Getting Ready" steps. ☐ ☐ _____

Procedure

2. Make sure that the bed is positioned at a comfortable working height (to promote good body mechanics) and that the wheels are locked. ☐ ☐ _____

3. Place the pillow at the head of the bed, on its edge against the headboard. This gets the pillow out of the way. It also pads the headboard in case you move the person up a little too much or too fast! ☐ ☐ _____

4. If the side rails are in use, lower the side rails. Lower the head of the bed so that the bed is flat (as tolerated). Fanfold the top linens to the foot of the bed. ☐ ☐ _____

5. If the lift sheet is already on the bed, make sure that it is positioned so that it is under the person's shoulders and hips. (If a lift sheet is not already on the bed, position one under the person's shoulders and hips.) ☐ ☐ _____

6. Stand at the side of the bed, opposite your co-worker, with your feet spread about 12 inches apart and with your knees slightly bent to protect your back. ☐ ☐ _____

7. Grasp the edge of the lift sheet and roll it over as close to the person's body as possible. This will provide for a better grip. (Your co-worker does the same.) ☐ ☐ _____

8. Grasp the rolled edge of the lift sheet with both hands, palms and fingers facing down. One hand should be level with the person's shoulders and the other should be level with his or her hips. ☐ ☐ _____

9. On the count of "three," slowly and carefully lift up on the lift sheet in unison and move the person toward the head of the bed. Avoid dragging the person across the bottom linens. ☐ ☐ _____

10. Reposition the pillow under the person's head and straighten the bottom linens. Draw the top linens over the person. Raise the head of the bed as the person requests. ☐ ☐ _____

11. Make sure that the bed is lowered to its lowest position and that the wheels are locked. If the side rails are in use, return them to the raised position. ☐ ☐ _____

Finishing Up

12. Complete the "Finishing Up" steps. ☐ ☐ _____

PROCEDURE 14-5
Turning a Person Onto His or Her Side

	S	U	COMMENTS

Getting Ready

1. Complete the "Getting Ready" steps.   ☐ ☐ _____

Procedure

2. Make sure that the bed is positioned at a comfortable working height (to promote good body mechanics) and that the wheels are locked.   ☐ ☐ _____

3. Place the pillow at the head of the bed, on its edge against the headboard. This gets the pillow out of the way.   ☐ ☐ _____

4. If the side rails are in use, lower the side rail on the working side of the bed. The side rail on the opposite side of the bed should remain up. Lower the head of the bed so that the bed is flat (as tolerated). Fanfold the top linens to the foot of the bed.   ☐ ☐ _____

5. Stand at the side of the bed with your feet spread about 12 inches apart and with your knees slightly bent to protect your back.   ☐ ☐ _____

6. Move the person to the side of the bed nearest you.   ☐ ☐ _____

7. Cross the person's arm that is nearest you over the person's chest.   ☐ ☐ _____

8. Bend the person's leg that is nearest you, placing the foot on the bed. (Or, cross the person's leg that is nearest to you over her other leg.)   ☐ ☐ _____

9. Roll the person onto her side:

   a. **To roll the person away from you:** Place one of your hands on the person's shoulder that is nearest you, and place your other hand on the person's hip that is nearest you. Gently roll the person away from you, toward the opposite side of the bed.   ☐ ☐ _____

   b. **To roll the person toward you:** Raise the side rail and move to the other side of the bed. Lower that side rail. Place one hand on the person's shoulder that is farthest away from you, and place your other hand on the person's hip that is farthest away from you. Gently roll the person toward you.   ☐ ☐ _____

10. Reposition the pillow under the person's head and straighten the bottom linens. Support the person by placing a pillow lengthwise between the person's legs. The person's lower leg should be straight, and the upper leg should be slightly bent at the knee. Place additional pillows under the person's upper arm, and behind her back. Draw the top linens over the person.   ☐ ☐ _____

11. Make sure that the bed is lowered to its lowest position and that the wheels are locked. If the side rails are in use, return them to the raised position. ☐ ☐ _____

Finishing Up

12. Complete the "Finishing Up" steps. ☐ ☐ _____

PROCEDURE 14-6
Logrolling a Person (Two Assistants)

	S	U	COMMENTS

Getting Ready

1. Complete the "Getting Ready" steps.   ☐ ☐ _____

Procedure

2. Make sure that the bed is positioned at a comfortable working height (to promote good body mechanics) and that the wheels are locked.   ☐ ☐ _____

3. Place the pillow at the head of the bed, on its edge against the headboard. This gets the pillow out of the way.   ☐ ☐ _____

4. If the side rails are in use, lower the side rail on the working side of the bed. The side rail on the opposite side of the bed should remain up. Lower the head of the bed so that the bed is flat (as tolerated). Fanfold the top linens to the foot of the bed.   ☐ ☐ _____

5. Stand with the other assistant on the side of the bed with the lowered side rail. Stand facing the bed with your feet spread about 12 inches apart and with your knees slightly bent to protect your back. One assistant is aligned with the person's head and shoulders; the other is aligned with the person's hips.   ☐ ☐ _____

6. Place your hands under the person's head and shoulders while your co-worker places his hands under the person's hips and legs (or vice versa). Lifting in unison, gently move the person toward the side of the bed closest to you.   ☐ ☐ _____

7. Place a pillow lengthwise between the person's legs and fold the person's arm so that it will be on top of his chest when he is turned.   ☐ ☐ _____

8. Raise the side rail and make sure that it is secure.   ☐ ☐ _____

9. Go to the opposite side of the bed and lower the side rail.   ☐ ☐ _____

10. Working with the other assistant, turn the person onto his side.

     a. If a lift sheet is being used, turn the person by reaching over him and grasping the lift sheet. One assistant should place one hand on the lift sheet at the level of the person's shoulder and the other hand at the level of the person's hip; the other assistant should place one hand on the lift sheet at the level of the person's hip and the other at the level of the person's calves.   ☐ ☐ _____

     b. If a lift sheet is not being used, one assistant should position her hands on the person's shoulders and hips and the other assistant should place his hands on the person's thigh and calves.   ☐ ☐ _____

11. On the count of "three," roll the person toward
    the side on which you are standing in a single
    movement, being sure to keep the person's head,
    spine, and legs aligned. ☐ ☐ _____

12. Reposition the pillow under the person's head and
    straighten the bottom linens. Support the person by
    bolstering his back with pillows. The pillow between
    the person's legs should remain in place, and
    additional pillows or folded towels should be used to
    support the person's arms. Draw the top linens over
    the person. ☐ ☐ _____

13. Make sure that the bed is lowered to its lowest
    position and that the wheels are locked. If the side
    rails are in use, return them to the raised position. ☐ ☐ _____

Finishing Up

14. Complete the "Finishing Up" steps. ☐ ☐ _____

PROCEDURE 14-7

Assisting a Person With Sitting on the Edge of the Bed ("Dangling")

	S	U	COMMENTS

Getting Ready

1. Complete the "Getting Ready" steps. ☐ ☐ _____

Procedure

2. Make sure that the bed is lowered to its lowest position and that the wheels are locked. ☐ ☐ _____

3. If the side rails are in use, lower the side rail on the working side of the bed. The side rail on the opposite side of the bed should remain up. Raise the head of the bed as tolerated. Fanfold the top linens to the foot of the bed. ☐ ☐ _____

4. **Method "A":**

   a. Stand at the side of the bed with your feet spread about 12 inches apart and with your knees slightly bent to protect your back. ☐ ☐ _____

   b. Have the person bend her knees and plant her feet on the bed. ☐ ☐ _____

   c. Gently slide one arm behind the person's upper back. Slide the other arm under her knees and rest your hand on the side of her thigh. ☐ ☐ _____

   d. With a single smooth movement, slide the person's legs over the side of the bed while moving her head and shoulders upward so that she is sitting on the edge of the bed. ☐ ☐ _____

5. **Method "B":**

   a. Help the person to move toward the side of the bed. ☐ ☐ _____

   b. Have the person roll over onto her side, facing the side of the bed. Have the person flex her knees and bend the arm she is lying on in preparation for using it to prop her upper body up. Have the person bend her top arm so that her hand is in a position that will enable her to push off the bed. ☐ ☐ _____

   c. Instruct the person to rise to a sitting position by using the elbow of her bottom arm to raise her upper body while pushing against the mattress with her other hand. Advise the person to allow her legs to swing over the edge of the bed while you help to guide her into an upright position. ☐ ☐ _____

6. Have the person put her hands on the edge of the bed, alongside each thigh, for support. Watch for signs of dizziness or fainting. If the person feels faint, help her to lie down and call for the nurse. ☐ ☐ _____

7. Allow the person to "dangle" her legs over the side of the bed for the specified period of time, and then either take her vital signs (if indicated), help her to lie back down, or assist her to a standing position. Stay with her during the entire time. ☐ ☐ _____

Finishing Up

8. Complete the "Finishing Up" steps. ☐ ☐ _____

PROCEDURE 14-8
Applying a Transfer (Gait) Belt

	S	U	COMMENTS

Getting Ready

1. Complete the "Getting Ready" steps.   ☐ ☐ _____

Procedure

2. If the person is in bed, make sure that the bed is lowered to its lowest position and that the wheels are locked. If the side rails are in use, lower the side rail on the working side of the bed. The side rail on the opposite side of the bed should remain up. Fanfold the top linens to the foot of the bed. Assist the person to sit on the edge of the bed.   ☐ ☐ _____

3. Apply the belt around the person's waist, over her clothing. Buckle the belt in the front by threading the tongue of the belt through the side of the buckle that has "teeth" first, and then placing the tongue of the belt through the other side of the buckle.   ☐ ☐ _____

4. Before tightening the belt, turn it so that the buckle is off-center in the front or to the side.   ☐ ☐ _____

5. Tighten the belt and check for fit. The belt should be snug, but you should be able to slip your fingers between the belt and the person's waist. When applying a transfer belt to a woman, make sure that her breasts are not trapped underneath the belt.   ☐ ☐ _____

6. Use an underhand grasp when holding the belt to provide greater safety.   ☐ ☐ _____

Finishing Up

7. When the person has finished transferring and is ready to return to bed, reverse the procedure.   ☐ ☐ _____

8. Complete the "Finishing Up" steps.   ☐ ☐ _____

PROCEDURE 14-9

Transferring a Person From a Bed to a Wheelchair (One Assistant)

	S	U	COMMENTS
Getting Ready			
1. Complete the "Getting Ready" steps.	☐	☐	_____

Procedure

	S	U	COMMENTS
2. Determine the person's strongest side, and then place the wheelchair alongside the bed. Position the wheelchair so that the person will move toward the chair "strong side first." Whenever possible, position the wheelchair so that it is against a wall or a solid piece of furniture so that it will not slide backward during the transfer.	☐	☐	_____
3. Lock the wheelchair wheels, and either remove the footrests or swing them to the side.	☐	☐	_____
4. Fanfold the top linens to the foot of the bed.	☐	☐	_____
5. Make sure that the bed is lowered to its lowest position and that the wheels are locked. Raise the head of the bed as tolerated.	☐	☐	_____
6. Help the person to move toward the side of the bed where the wheelchair is located.	☐	☐	_____
7. Assist the person to dangle.	☐	☐	_____
8. Allow the person to rest on the edge of the bed. The person should be sitting squarely on both buttocks, with her knees apart and both feet flat on the floor (to offer a broad base of support). The person's arms should rest alongside her thighs. Watch for signs of dizziness or fainting. Position yourself in front of the person so that you can offer assistance in case she loses balance.	☐	☐	_____
9. Help the person to put her shoes or slippers on and help her to get into a robe. Apply a transfer belt.	☐	☐	_____
10. Help the person to stand.			
a. Stand facing the person.	☐	☐	_____
b. Have the person put her hands on the edge of the bed, alongside each thigh.	☐	☐	_____
c. Make sure the person's feet are flat on the floor.	☐	☐	_____
d. Have the person lean forward.	☐	☐	_____
e. Grasp the transfer belt at each side, using an underhand grasp. (If you are not using a transfer belt, pass your arms under the person's arms and rest your hands on her upper back.)	☐	☐	_____
f. Position your feet alongside the person's feet, flexing your knees. Place your shins against the person's shins to block the person's feet and keep her knees from buckling as she stands up.	☐	☐	_____

g. Have the person push down on the bed with her hands and stand on the count of "three." Assist the person into a standing position by pulling on the transfer belt as you straighten your knees. (If you are not using a transfer belt, assist the person into a standing position by gently pulling her up and forward as you straighten your knees.) Remember to keep your back straight. □ □ _____

11. Support the person in the standing position by holding the transfer belt or by keeping your hands on her upper back. Continue to block the person's feet and knees with your feet and knees. □ □ _____

12. Help the person to turn by pivoting on the stronger leg toward the chair. This will allow the person to grasp the far arm of the wheelchair. □ □ _____

13. Continue to assist the person with turning until she is able to grasp the other armrest. The backs of the person's legs should touch the edge of the chair. □ □ _____

14. Lower the person into the wheelchair by bending your hips and knees. □ □ _____

15. Make sure the person's buttocks are at the back of the chair. Make sure the person is comfortable and in good body alignment. □ □ _____

16. Remove the transfer belt. □ □ _____

17. Position the person's feet on the footrests of the wheelchair. Buckle the wheelchair safety belt (if ordered) and cover the person's lap and legs with a lap blanket, if desired. Make sure that the lap blanket does not drag on the floor. □ □ _____

Finishing Up

18. Position the wheelchair according to the person's preference. □ □ _____

19. Complete the "Finishing Up" steps. □ □ _____

PROCEDURE 14-10

Transferring a Person From a Bed to a Wheelchair (Two Assistants)

	S	U	COMMENTS

Getting Ready

1. Complete the "Getting Ready" steps. ☐ ☐ _____

Procedure

2. Place the wheelchair alongside the bed, facing the foot of the bed. ☐ ☐ _____

3. Lock the wheelchair wheels and either remove the footrests or swing them to the side. ☐ ☐ _____

4. Fanfold the top linens to the foot of the bed. ☐ ☐ _____

5. Make sure that the bed is positioned at a comfortable working height (to promote good body mechanics) and that the wheels are locked. Raise the head of the bed as tolerated. ☐ ☐ _____

6. Help the person to move toward the side of the bed where the wheelchair is located. ☐ ☐ _____

7. Help the person to put his shoes or slippers on, and help him get into a robe. ☐ ☐ _____

8. Stand by the side of the bed, behind the wheelchair. Standing behind the person, pass your arms under the person's arms and grasp his forearms. The other assistant grasps the person's thighs and calves. ☐ ☐ _____

9. Working in unison with the other assistant, lift the person from the bed and bring him toward the wheelchair on the count of "three." Lower the person into the wheelchair. ☐ ☐ _____

10. Make sure the person's buttocks are at the back of the chair. Make sure the person is comfortable and in good body alignment. ☐ ☐ _____

11. Position the person's feet on the footrests of the wheelchair. Buckle the wheelchair safety belt (if ordered) and cover the person's lap and legs with a lap blanket, if desired. Make sure that the lap blanket does not drag on the floor. ☐ ☐ _____

Finishing Up

12. Position the wheelchair according to the person's preference. ☐ ☐ _____

13. Complete the "Finishing Up" steps. ☐ ☐ _____

PROCEDURE 14-11

Transferring a Person From a Wheelchair to a Bed

	S	U	COMMENTS

Getting Ready

1. Complete the "Getting Ready" steps. □ □ _____

Procedure

2. Make sure that the bed is lowered to its lowest position and that the wheels are locked. Raise the head of the bed, fanfold the top linens to the foot of the bed, and raise the opposite side rail. □ □ _____

3. Position the wheelchair close to the side of the bed so that the person's strong side is next to the bed. Lock the wheelchair wheels and either remove the footrests or swing them to the side. □ □ _____

4. Remove the person's lap blanket (if one was used) and release the wheelchair safety belt, if in use. Apply a transfer belt. □ □ _____

5. Stand facing the person with your feet spread about 12 inches apart and with your knees slightly bent to protect your back. With your back straight, slide the person to the front of the wheelchair seat. □ □ _____

6. Grasp the transfer belt (or pass your arms under the person's arms, placing your hands on her upper back). Position your feet alongside the person's feet, flexing your knees. Place your shins against the person's shins to block the person's feet and keep her knees from buckling as she stands up. □ □ _____

7. Have the person rest her hands on your arms and assist her to stand by pulling on the transfer belt as you straighten your knees. (If you are not using a transfer belt, assist the person into a standing position by gently pulling her up and forward as you straighten your knees.) Remember to keep your back straight. Alternatively, a person who requires less assistance can place her hands on the wheelchair arms for support and "push off" while you offer support. □ □ _____

8. Slowly help the person to turn toward the bed by pivoting on her strong leg. Help the person to sit on the edge of the bed. □ □ _____

9. Remove the person's robe and slippers, if appropriate. □ □ _____

10. Move the wheelchair out of the way. □ □ _____

11. Place one of your arms around the person's shoulders and one arm under her legs. Swing the person's legs onto the bed. □ □ _____

12. Help the person to move to the center of the bed and position her comfortably. □ □ _____

13. Straighten the bottom linens and make sure the person is comfortable and in good body alignment. Draw the top linens over the person.   ☐ ☐ _____

14. If the side rails are in use, return them to the raised position.   ☐ ☐ _____

Finishing Up

15. Complete the "Finishing Up" steps.   ☐ ☐ _____

PROCEDURE 14-12
Transferring a Person From a Bed to a Stretcher (Four Assistants)

	S	U	COMMENTS

Getting Ready

1. Complete the "Getting Ready" steps. ☐ ☐ _____

Procedure

2. Raise the bed to its highest level. (The stretcher should be slightly lower than the bed.) Lower the head of the bed so that the bed is flat. Make sure that the bed wheels are locked. Lower the side rails. Fanfold the top linens to the side of the bed opposite the stretcher. ☐ ☐ _____

3. If the lift sheet is already on the bed, make sure that it is positioned so that it is under the person's shoulders and hips. (If a lift sheet is not already on the bed, position one under the person's shoulders and hips.) ☐ ☐ _____

4. Position the stretcher alongside the bed. Lock the stretcher wheels and move the stretcher safety belts out of the way. ☐ ☐ _____

5. Two assistants stand at the side of the bed facing their co-workers, who are positioned along the outside edge of the stretcher. ☐ ☐ _____

6. Grasp the edge of the lift sheet and roll it over as close to the person's body as possible. This will provide for a better grip. (Your co-workers do the same.) ☐ ☐ _____

7. On the count of "three," all four assistants slowly and carefully lift up on the lift sheet in unison and move the person to the side of the bed. ☐ ☐ _____

8. On the count of "three," all four assistants slowly and carefully lift up on the transfer sheet in unison and move the person to the side of the stretcher. ☐ ☐ _____

9. Position the person on the stretcher and make sure he is in good body alignment. Reposition the pillow under the person's head and cover the person with a blanket for modesty and warmth. Buckle the stretcher safety belts across the person and raise the side rails on the stretcher. Raise the head of the stretcher as the person requests. ☐ ☐ _____

Finishing Up

10. Transport the person to the appropriate site. A person on a stretcher should always be transported "feet first." Remain with the person; never leave someone alone on a stretcher. ☐ ☐ _____

11. Complete the "Finishing Up" steps. ☐ ☐ _____

PROCEDURE 14-13

Transferring a Person From a Stretcher to a Bed (Four Assistants)

Getting Ready	S	U	COMMENTS
1. Complete the "Getting Ready" steps.	☐	☐	_____

Procedure

	S	U	COMMENTS
2. Raise or lower the bed so that it is slightly lower than the stretcher. Lower the head of the bed so that the bed is flat. Make sure that the bed wheels are locked. Lower the side rails. Fanfold the top linens to the side of the bed opposite the stretcher.	☐	☐	_____
3. If the lift sheet is already on the stretcher, make sure that it is positioned so that it is under the person's shoulders and hips. (If a lift sheet is not already on the stretcher, position one under the person's shoulders and hips.)	☐	☐	_____
4. Unbuckle the stretcher safety belts and lower the side rails on the stretcher.	☐	☐	_____
5. Position the stretcher against the bed and lock the stretcher wheels.	☐	☐	_____
6. Two assistants stand at the far side of the bed facing their co-workers, who are positioned along the outside edge of the stretcher. (Some facilities allow the assistants on the far side of the bed to kneel on the bed to complete the transfer; follow your facility's policy.)	☐	☐	_____
7. Grasp the edge of the lift sheet and roll it over as close to the person's body as possible. This will provide for a better grip. (Your co-workers do the same.)	☐	☐	_____
8. On the count of "three," all four assistants slowly and carefully lift up on the lift sheet in unison and move the person to the bed. Move the stretcher away from the bed.	☐	☐	_____
9. Help the person to move to the center of the bed and, if desired, remove the lift sheet by turning the person first to one side, then the other. Position the person comfortably.	☐	☐	_____
10. Straighten the bottom linens and make sure the person is comfortable and in good body alignment. Draw the top linens over the person.	☐	☐	_____
11. Make sure the bed is lowered to its lowest position and that the wheels are locked. If the side rails are in use, return them to the raised position.	☐	☐	_____

Finishing Up

	S	U	COMMENTS
12. Complete the "Finishing Up" steps.	☐	☐	_____

PROCEDURE 14-14
Transferring a Person Using a Mechanical Lift (Two Assistants)

	S	U	COMMENTS

Getting Ready

1. Complete the "Getting Ready" steps. ☐ ☐ _____

Procedure

2. Make sure that the bed is positioned at a comfortable working height (to promote good body mechanics) and that the wheels are locked. ☐ ☐ _____

3. If the side rails are in use, lower the side rails. ☐ ☐ _____

4. Fanfold the top linens to the foot of the bed. ☐ ☐ _____

5. Center the sling under the person. (To get the sling under the person, move the person as if you were making an occupied bed.) The lower edge of the sling should be positioned underneath the person's knees. ☐ ☐ _____

6. Raise the head of the bed as tolerated. ☐ ☐ _____

7. Move the release valve on the lift to the closed position. ☐ ☐ _____

8. Raise the lift so that it can be positioned over the person. ☐ ☐ _____

9. Spread the legs of the lift to provide a solid base of support. The legs must be locked in this position, or the lift could tip over, injuring you, the person you are trying to transfer, or both. ☐ ☐ _____

10. Move the lift into position over the person. ☐ ☐ _____

11. Fasten the sling to the straps or chains of the lift. Make sure the hooks face away from the person. ☐ ☐ _____

12. Attach the sling to the swivel bar with the short side attached to the top of the sling and the long side attached to the bottom of the sling. ☐ ☐ _____

13. Cross the person's arms across her chest. The person may hold onto the straps, but do not let her hold onto the swivel bar. ☐ ☐ _____

14. Raise the lift until the person and the sling are clear of the bed. ☐ ☐ _____

15. Place the wheelchair alongside the bed, facing the foot of the bed. Lock the wheelchair wheels. ☐ ☐ _____

16. Have your co-worker support the person's legs as you move the lift into position over the wheelchair. ☐ ☐ _____

17. Turn the person so that she is facing the mast of the lift and is centered over the base. (The person's back should be facing the wheelchair.) ☐ ☐ _____

18. Move the lift so that the person is over the seat of the wheelchair. ☐ ☐ _____

19. Slowly open the release valve on the lift. Gently lower the person into the wheelchair. Make sure the person's buttocks are at the back of the chair. ☐ ☐ _____

20. Lower the swivel bar so that you can unhook the sling. Leave the sling under the person. ☐ ☐ _____

21. Make sure the person's buttocks are at the back of the chair. Make sure the person is comfortable and in good body alignment. ☐ ☐ _____

22. Position the person's feet on the footrests of the wheelchair. Buckle the wheelchair safety belt (or place a lap restraint, if ordered). Cover the person's lap and legs with a lap blanket, if desired. Make sure that the lap blanket does not drag on the floor. ☐ ☐ _____

Finishing Up

23. Position the wheelchair according to the person's preference. ☐ ☐ _____

24. Follow the "Finishing Up" steps. ☐ ☐ _____

25. When the person is ready to return to bed, reverse the procedure. ☐ ☐ _____

CHAPTER 15 PROCEDURE CHECKLISTS

PROCEDURE 15-1
Assisting a Person With Walking (Ambulating)

Getting Ready	S	U	COMMENTS
1. Complete the "Getting Ready" steps.	☐	☐	_____

Procedure

	S	U	COMMENTS
2. If the person is in bed, make sure that the bed is lowered to its lowest position and that the wheels are locked.	☐	☐	_____
3. Assist the person to "dangle." Check the person's pulse; a weak pulse could lead to lightheadedness. If the person's pulse is weak, stay with her and alert the nurse before attempting ambulation.	☐	☐	_____
4. Help the person put her shoes or slippers on and help her into a robe. Apply a transfer belt.	☐	☐	_____
5. Help the person to stand.			
a. Stand facing the person.	☐	☐	_____
b. Have the person put her hands on the edge of the bed, alongside each thigh.	☐	☐	_____
c. Make sure the person's feet are flat on the floor.	☐	☐	_____
d. Have the person lean forward.	☐	☐	_____
e. Grasp the transfer belt at each side, using an underhand grasp. (If you are not using a transfer belt, pass your arms under the person's arms and rest your hands on her upper back.)	☐	☐	_____
f. Position your feet alongside the person's feet, flexing your knees. Place your shins against the person's shins to block the person's feet and keep her knees from buckling as she stands up.	☐	☐	_____
g. Have the person push down on the bed with her hands and stand on the count of "three." Assist the person into a standing position by pulling on the transfer belt as you straighten your knees. (If you are not using a transfer belt, assist the person into a standing position by gently pulling her up and forward as you straighten your knees.) Remember to keep your back straight.	☐	☐	_____
6. Have the person grasp the cane or walker, if she is using one, in order to maintain balance. The person should hold the cane on her strong side.	☐	☐	_____
7. Help the person to walk. Stand slightly behind the person on her weaker side. Grasp the transfer belt with an underhand grip from the back. If the person is using an ambulation device, make sure she is using it correctly.	☐	☐	_____

8. After returning to the person's room, help her back into bed or a chair.   ☐ ☐ _____

Finishing Up

9. Complete the "Finishing Up" steps.   ☐ ☐ _____

PROCEDURE 15-2
Assisting a Person With Passive Range-of-Motion Exercises

	S	U	COMMENTS

Getting Ready

1. Complete the "Getting Ready" steps. ☐ ☐ _____

Procedure

2. Make sure that the bed is positioned at a comfortable ☐ ☐ _____
   working height (to promote good body mechanics)
   and that the wheels are locked. If the side rails are in
   use, lower the side rail on the working side of the
   bed. The side rail on the opposite side of the bed
   should remain up. Raise or lower the head of the bed
   to a horizontal or semi-Fowler's position.

3. Assist the person into the supine position. ☐ ☐ _____

4. Spread the bath blanket over the top linens (and the ☐ ☐ _____
   person). If the person is able, have him hold the bath
   blanket. If not, tuck the corners under his shoulders.
   Fanfold the top linens to the foot of the bed.

5. Perform each range-of-motion exercise in steps 6 ☐ ☐ _____
   through 13 according to the person's care plan, being
   careful to expose only the part of the body that is
   being exercised. Repeat each exercise three to five
   times, as written in the care plan.

6. If your facility permits, exercise the person's neck:

   a. Forward and backward flexion and extension ☐ ☐ _____
      (neck). Support the person's head by putting one
      hand under his chin and the other on the back of
      the head. Gently bring the head forward, as if to
      touch the chin to the chest, and then bring it
      backward, chin pointing to the sky.

   b. Side-to-side flexion (neck). Support the person's ☐ ☐ _____
      head by putting one hand under his chin and the
      other near the opposite temple. Gently tilt the
      head toward the right shoulder and then toward
      the left.

   c. Rotation (neck). Support the person's head by ☐ ☐ _____
      putting one hand under his chin and the other
      on the back of the head. Gently move the head
      from side to side, as if the person were shaking
      his head "no."

7. Exercise the person's shoulder:

   a. Forward flexion and extension (shoulder). Support ☐ ☐ _____
      the person's arm by putting one hand under his
      elbow and the other under his wrist. Keeping the
      person's arm straight with the palm facing down,
      lift the arm up so that it is alongside his ear and
      then return it to its original position.

b. Abduction and adduction (shoulder). Support the person's arm by putting one hand under his elbow and the other under his wrist. Keeping the person's arm straight with the palm facing up, move his arm away from the side of his body and then return it to its original position. ☐ ☐ _____

c. Horizontal abduction and adduction (shoulder). Support the person's arm by putting one hand under his elbow and the other under his wrist. Keeping the person's arm straight with the palm facing up, move his arm away from the side of his body. Gently bending the person's elbow, touch his hand to the opposite shoulder, then straighten the elbow and bring the arm back out to the side. ☐ ☐ _____

d. Rotation (shoulder). Support the person's arm by putting one hand under his elbow and the other under his wrist. Move the person's arm away from the side of his body and bend his arm at the elbow. Gently move the person's forearm up so that it forms a right angle with the mattress and then back down. This movement is similar to the motion a police officer makes when he is signaling someone to stop. ☐ ☐ _____

8. Exercise the person's elbow.

a. Flexion and extension (elbow). Support the person's arm by putting one hand under his elbow and the other under his wrist. Starting with the person's arm straight and with the palm facing up, bend his elbow so that his hand moves toward his shoulder. Then, straighten out the elbow, returning the person's hand to its original position. ☐ ☐ _____

b. Pronation and supination (elbow). Support the person's arm by putting one hand under his elbow and the other under his wrist. Move the person's arm away from the side of his body and slightly bend his arm at the elbow. Gently move the person's forearm up so that it forms a right angle with the mattress. Gently turn the person's hand so that the palm is facing the end of the bed. Then turn the hand the other way so that the palm is facing the head of the bed. ☐ ☐ _____

9. Exercise the person's wrist.

a. Flexion and extension (wrist). Support the person's wrist with one hand. Use the other hand to gently bend the person's hand down and then back. ☐ ☐ _____

b. Radial and ulnar flexion (wrist). Support the person's wrist with one hand. Use the other hand to gently turn the person's hand toward his thumb. Then turn the hand the other way, toward the little finger. ☐ ☐ _____

10. Exercise the person's fingers and thumb.

    a. Flexion and extension (fingers and thumb). Support the person's wrist with one hand. Using your other hand, flex the person's fingers to make a fist, tucking his thumb under the fingers. Then straighten each finger and the thumb, one by one. ☐ ☐ _____

    b. Abduction and adduction (fingers and thumb). With one hand, hold the person's thumb and index finger together. With the other hand, move the middle finger away from the index finger. Then move the middle finger back toward the index finger and hold the middle finger, index finger and thumb together. Next, move the ring finger away from the other two fingers and thumb, then move it back toward the group. Do the same with the little finger. Finally, reverse the process. Hold the little finger and the ring finger together and move the middle finger away and back. Complete with the index finger and thumb. ☐ ☐ _____

    c. Flexion and extension (thumb). Bend the person's thumb into his palm, then return it to its original position. ☐ ☐ _____

    d. Opposition. Touch each fingertip to the thumb. ☐ ☐ _____

11. Exercise the person's hip and knee.

    a. Forward flexion and extension (hip and knee). Support the person's leg by putting one hand under his knee and the other under his ankle. Gently bend the person's knee, moving it toward his head. Then straighten the person's knee and gently lower the leg to the bed. ☐ ☐ _____

    b. Abduction and adduction (hip). Support the person's leg by putting one hand under his knee and the other under his ankle. Keeping the person's leg straight, move his leg away from the side of his body and then return it to its original position. ☐ ☐ _____

    c. Rotation (hip). Support the person's leg by putting one hand under his knee and the other under his ankle. Keeping the person's leg straight, gently turn the leg inward and then outward. ☐ ☐ _____

12. Exercise the person's ankle and foot.

    a. Dorsiflexion and plantar flexion (ankle and foot). Support the person's ankle with one hand. Use the other hand to gently bend the person's foot up toward the head and then back. ☐ ☐ _____

    b. Inversion and eversion (ankle and foot). Support the person's ankle with one hand. Use the other hand to gently turn the inside of the foot inward and then outward. ☐ ☐ _____

13. Exercise the person's toes.

   a. Flexion and extension (toes). Put one hand under the person's foot. Put the other hand over the person's toes. Curl the toes downward and then straighten them.   ☐ ☐ _____

   b. Abduction and adduction (toes). Spread each toe the same way you spread each finger in step 10b.   ☐ ☐ _____

14. Straighten the bed linens and make sure the person is comfortable and in good body alignment. Draw the top linens over the person and remove the bath blanket.   ☐ ☐ _____

15. If the side rails are in use, raise the side rail on the working side of the bed. Make sure that the bed is lowered to its lowest position and that the wheels are locked.   ☐ ☐ _____

Finishing Up

16. Complete the "Finishing Up" steps.   ☐ ☐ _____

CHAPTER 16 PROCEDURE CHECKLISTS

PROCEDURE 16-1
Making an Unoccupied (Closed) Bed

Getting Ready	S	U	COMMENTS
1. Complete the "Getting Ready" steps.	☐	☐	

Procedure

	S	U	COMMENTS
2. Place the linens on a clean surface close to the bed (e.g., the over-bed table).	☐	☐	
3. Make sure that the bed is positioned at a comfortable working height (to promote good body mechanics) and that the wheels are locked.	☐	☐	
4. Lower the side rails and move the mattress to the head of the bed (it may have shifted toward the foot of the bed if the occupant of the bed had the head of the bed elevated).	☐	☐	

Note: The mattress pad, bottom sheet, and draw sheet are positioned and tucked in on one side of the bed before moving to the other side to complete these actions. This is most efficient in terms of energy and time.

	S	U	COMMENTS
5. Place the mattress pad on the bed and unfold it so that only one vertical crease remains. Make sure that this crease is centered on the mattress. If the mattress pad is fitted, carefully pull the corners of the near side over the corners of the mattress and smooth down the sides. If the mattress pad is flat, make sure the top of the pad is even with the head of the mattress. Open the mattress pad across the bed, taking care to keep it centered.	☐	☐	

6. Place the bottom sheet on the bed. If the bottom sheet is fitted, carefully pull the corners of the near side over the corners of the mattress and smooth down the sides. If the bottom sheet is flat:

	S	U	COMMENTS
a. Place the sheet so that when you unfold it, the wide hem will be at the head of the bed and the hem stitching will be against the mattress, away from the person who will be occupying the bed.	☐	☐	
b. Unfold the sheet so that only one vertical crease remains. Make sure that this crease is vertically centered on the mattress.	☐	☐	
c. Open the sheet across the bed, taking care to keep it centered. The same length of sheet (approximately 12 to 18 inches) should hang over each side of the bed. Make sure that the lower edge of the sheet is even with the foot of the mattress.	☐	☐	

d. Tuck the sheet under the mattress at the head of the bed and miter the corner. ☐ ☐ _____

e. Tuck the near side of the sheet underneath the mattress, working from the head of the bed toward the foot. As you tuck, make sure there are no wrinkles in the sheet and that the mattress pad remains smooth and in place. ☐ ☐ _____

7. Place the lift sheet on the bed so that the top of the sheet is approximately 12 inches from the head of the mattress. If you are using a plastic or rubberized lift sheet, place a cotton lift sheet on top of it. Smooth the lift sheet across the bed and tuck the near side under the mattress. ☐ ☐ _____

8. Now, move to the other side of the bed and repeat the process of aligning the mattress pad, mitering the corner, and tucking in the bottom sheet and lift sheet. ☐ ☐ _____

9. Place the top sheet on the bed so that when you unfold it, the wide hem will be at the head of the bed and the hem stitching will be facing upward, away from the person who will be occupying the bed.

a. Unfold the sheet so that only one vertical crease remains. Make sure that this crease is centered vertically on the mattress. ☐ ☐ _____

b. Open the sheet across the bed, taking care to keep it centered. The same length of sheet (approximately 12 to 18 inches) should hang over each side of the bed. Make sure that the top edge of the sheet is even with the head of the mattress. Pull the bottom of the sheet over the foot of the bed, but do not tuck it in yet (it will be tucked in with the blanket and bedspread). ☐ ☐ _____

10. Place the blanket on the bed and unfold it in the same manner as the sheet, keeping the center crease in the center of the bed. The same length of blanket (approximately 12 to 18 inches) should hang over each side of the bed. Make sure that the top edge of the blanket is approximately 6 to 8 inches from the head of the mattress. Fold the top edge of the sheet back over the top edge of the blanket, creating a cuff. Pull the bottom edge of the blanket over the sheet at the foot of the bed, but do not tuck anything in yet. ☐ ☐ _____

11. Place the bedspread on the bed and unfold it in the same manner as the sheet, keeping the center crease in the center of the bed. The sides of the bedspread should be even and cover all of the other bed linens. Make sure that the top of the bedspread is even with the head of the mattress, unless the pillow is to be tucked under the bedspread (in which case you will need to allow more length at the top). Pull the bottom of the bedspread over the blanket and sheet at the foot of the bed. ☐ ☐ _____

12. Together, tuck the bedspread, the blanket, and the top sheet under the foot of the mattress. Make a mitered corner at the foot of the bed on both sides. ☐ ☐ _____

13. Fold the top of the bedspread back over the blanket to make a cuff. ☐ ☐ _____

14. Rest the pillow on the bed. Grasping the closed end of the pillowcase, turn the pillowcase inside out over your hand and arm. Grasp the pillow through the pillowcase and pull the pillowcase down over the pillow. Make sure any tags or zippers are on the inside of the pillowcase. ☐ ☐ _____

15. Place the pillow on the bed with the open end of the pillowcase facing away from the door. ☐ ☐ _____

Finishing Up

16. Complete the "Finishing Up" steps. ☐ ☐ _____

PROCEDURE 16-2
Making an Occupied Bed

	S	U	COMMENTS

Getting Ready

1. Complete the "Getting Ready" steps. ☐ ☐ _____

Procedure

2. Place the linens on a clean surface close to the bed (e.g., the over-bed table). ☐ ☐ _____

3. Make sure that the bed is positioned at a comfortable working height (to promote good body mechanics) and that the wheels are locked. ☐ ☐ _____

4. Remove the call-light control and check the bed for dentures or any other personal items. ☐ ☐ _____

5. Lower the head of the bed so that the bed is flat (as tolerated). ☐ ☐ _____

6. Put on the gloves (the linens may be wet or soiled). ☐ ☐ _____

7. Remove the bedspread and blanket from the bed. If they are to be reused, fold them and place them on a clean surface, such as a chair. ☐ ☐ _____

8. Loosen the top sheet at the foot of the bed and spread a bath blanket over the top sheet (and the person). ☐ ☐ _____

9. If the person is able, have her hold the bath blanket. If not, tuck the corners under the person's shoulders. Remove the top sheet by pulling it out from underneath the bath blanket, being careful not to expose the person. ☐ ☐ _____

10. Place the top sheet in the linen hamper or linen bag. ☐ ☐ _____

11. If the side rails are in use, lower the side rail on the working side of the bed. The side rail on the opposite side of the bed should remain up. Turn the person onto her side so that she is facing away from you. Reposition the pillow under the person's head, and adjust the bath blanket to keep the person covered. ☐ ☐ _____

12. Loosen the lift sheet, bottom sheet, and (if necessary) the mattress pad. ☐ ☐ _____

13. Fanfold the bottom linens toward the person's back, tucking them slightly underneath her. ☐ ☐ _____

14. Straighten the mattress pad (if it is not being changed). If the mattress pad is being changed, place the clean mattress pad on the bed and unfold it so that only one vertical crease remains. Make sure that this crease is centered vertically on the mattress. If the mattress pad is fitted, carefully pull the corners of the near side over the corners of the mattress and smooth down the sides. If the mattress pad is flat, make sure the top of the pad is even with the head of the mattress. Fanfold the opposite side of the mattress pad close to the patient or resident. ☐ ☐ _____

15. Place the clean bottom sheet on the bed. If the bottom sheet is fitted, carefully pull the corners over the corners of the mattress and smooth down the sides. If the bottom sheet is flat:

   a. Place the sheet so that when you unfold it, the wide hem will be at the head of the bed and the hem stitching will be against the mattress, away from the person who will be occupying the bed. ☐ ☐ _____

   b. Unfold the sheet so that only one vertical crease remains. Make sure that this crease is centered vertically on the mattress. ☐ ☐ _____

   c. Open the sheet across the bed, taking care to keep it centered. The same length of sheet (approximately 12 to 18 inches) should hang over each side of the bed. Make sure that the lower edge of the sheet is even with the foot of the mattress. Fanfold the opposite side of the sheet close to the patient or resident. ☐ ☐ _____

   d. Tuck the sheet under the mattress at the head of the bed and miter the corner. ☐ ☐ _____

   e. Tuck the near side of the sheet underneath the mattress, working from the head of the bed toward the foot. As you tuck, make sure there are no wrinkles in the sheet and that the mattress pad remains smooth and in place. ☐ ☐ _____

16. Place the lift sheet on the bed so that the top of the sheet is approximately 12 inches from the head of the mattress. If you are using a plastic or rubberized lift sheet, place a cotton lift sheet on top of it. Fanfold the opposite side of the lift sheet close to the patient or resident. Smooth the lift sheet across the bed and tuck the near side under the mattress. ☐ ☐ _____

17. Raise the side rail on the working side of the bed. Help the person to roll toward you, over the folded linens. Reposition the pillow under the person's head and adjust the bath blanket to keep the person covered. ☐ ☐ _____

18. Move to the other side of the bed and lower the side rail. ☐ ☐ _____

19. Loosen and remove the soiled bottom linens and place them in the linen hamper or linen bag. Change your gloves if they become soiled. ☐ ☐ _____

20. Now, repeat the process of aligning the mattress pad, mitering the corner, and tucking in the bottom sheet and lift sheet. ☐ ☐ _____

21. Help the person to move to the center of the bed and position her comfortably. Raise the side rail on the working side of the bed. ☐ ☐ _____

22. Change the pillowcase and place the pillow under the person's head. ☐ ☐ _____

23. Place the clean top sheet over the person (who is still covered with the bath blanket), being careful not to cover her face. The sheet should be placed so that when you unfold it, the wide hem will be at the head of the bed and the hem stitching will be facing upward, away from the person who will be occupying the bed.

   a. Unfold the sheet so that only one vertical crease remains. Make sure that this crease is centered vertically on the mattress.   ☐ ☐ _____

   b. Open the sheet across the bed, taking care to keep it centered. The same length of sheet (approximately 12 to 18 inches) should hang over each side of the bed.   ☐ ☐ _____

   c. If the person is able, have her hold the top sheet. If not, tuck the corners under her shoulders. Remove the bath blanket by pulling it out from underneath the top sheet, being careful not to expose the person. Place the bath blanket in the linen hamper or linen bag.   ☐ ☐ _____

24. Place the blanket and then the bedspread over the top sheet. Together, tuck the bedspread, the blanket, and the top sheet under the foot of the mattress. Make a mitered corner at the foot of the bed on both sides.   ☐ ☐ _____

25. Make a toe pleat by grasping the top sheet, the blanket, and the bedspread over the person's feet and pulling the linens straight up. The toe pleat allows the person to move her feet and helps to relieve pressure on the feet from tightly tucked linens.   ☐ ☐ _____

26. Lower the bed to its lowest position and make sure that the wheels are locked. Raise the head of the bed as the person requests.   ☐ ☐ _____

27. Remove your gloves and dispose of them in a facility-approved waste container.   ☐ ☐ _____

Finishing Up

28. Complete "Finishing Up" steps.   ☐ ☐ _____

CHAPTER 17 PROCEDURE CHECKLISTS

PROCEDURE 17-1
Measuring an Oral Temperature (Glass or Electronic Thermometer)

Getting Ready	S	U	COMMENTS
1. Complete the "Getting Ready" steps.	☐	☐	_____

Procedure

	S	U	COMMENTS
2. Ask the person if she has eaten, consumed a beverage, chewed gum, or smoked within the last 15 minutes. If so, wait 15 to 30 minutes before proceeding (or follow facility policy).	☐	☐	_____
3. Prepare the thermometer.			
a. **Glass thermometer:** Run cool water over the thermometer to rinse away the disinfectant. Dry the thermometer with a paper towel and inspect it for cracks or chips. Carefully shake down the glass thermometer so that the indicator material is below the 94° mark (if using a Fahrenheit thermometer) or the 34° mark (if using a Celsius thermometer). Cover the end of the glass thermometer with the thermometer sheath.	☐	☐	_____
b. **Electronic thermometer:** Cover the electronic probe with the probe sheath. Turn the thermometer on and wait until the "ready" sign appears on the display screen.	☐	☐	_____
4. Ask the person to open her mouth. Slowly and carefully insert the thermometer, placing the tip under the person's tongue and to one side.	☐	☐	_____
5. Ask the person to gently close her mouth around the thermometer without biting down. If necessary, hold the thermometer in place. Ask the person to breathe through her nose.	☐	☐	_____
6. Leave the thermometer in place for the specified amount of time:			
a. **Glass thermometer:** 3 to 5 minutes (or follow facility policy)	☐	☐	_____
b. **Electronic thermometer:** until the instrument blinks or beeps (usually just a few seconds)	☐	☐	_____
7. Ask the person to open her mouth. Remove the thermometer from the person's mouth.	☐	☐	_____
8. Read the temperature measurement.			
a. **Glass thermometer:** Using a tissue, remove the thermometer sheath from the glass thermometer, being careful not to touch the bulb end of the thermometer. Dispose of the tissue and the thermometer sheath in a facility-approved waste	☐	☐	_____

container. Hold the thermometer horizontally by the stem at eye level while facing a light source. Rotate the thermometer until you can see the level of the indicator material. Read the temperature.

b. **Electronic thermometer:** Read the temperature on the electronic thermometer's display screen. Remove the probe sheath from the probe by pushing the button on the top of the probe. Direct the probe sheath into a facility-approved waste container.

☐ ☐ _____

9. Prepare the thermometer for its next use.

a. **Glass thermometer:** Shake down the glass thermometer, clean it according to facility policy, and return it to its disinfectant-filled case.

☐ ☐ _____

b. **Electronic thermometer:** Replace the probe into the electronic thermometer. (Always read the temperature before placing the probe in the instrument because this action clears the display screen.) Turn the instrument off if it does not automatically turn itself off. Place the thermometer in its charger.

☐ ☐ _____

10. Note the person's name, the time, the temperature, and the method on your notepad (or record the temperature and the method on the person's medical record if it is kept at the bedside). Place an "O" (or the notation designated by your facility) next to the measurement to indicate that the measurement was taken orally. Report an abnormal temperature to the nurse immediately.

☐ ☐ _____

Finishing Up

11. Complete the "Finishing Up" steps.

☐ ☐ _____

PROCEDURE 17-2

Measuring a Rectal Temperature (Glass or Electronic Thermometer)

Getting Ready	S	U	COMMENTS
1. Complete the "Getting Ready" steps.	☐	☐	_____

Procedure

	S	U	COMMENTS
2. Make sure that the bed is positioned at a comfortable working height (to promote good body mechanics) and that the wheels are locked.	☐	☐	_____
3. Prepare the thermometer.			
a. **Glass thermometer:** Run cool water over the thermometer to rinse away the disinfectant. Dry the thermometer with a paper towel and inspect it for cracks or chips. Carefully shake down the glass thermometer so that the indicator material is below the 94° mark (if using a Fahrenheit thermometer) or the 34° mark (if using a Celsius thermometer). Cover the end of the glass thermometer with the thermometer sheath.	☐	☐	_____
b. **Electronic thermometer:** Cover the electronic probe with the probe sheath. Turn the thermometer on and wait until the "ready" sign appears on the display screen.	☐	☐	_____
4. Place the thermometer on a clean paper towel on the over-bed table. Open the lubricant package and squeeze a small amount of lubricant onto the paper towel. Lubricate the tip of the thermometer to ease insertion.	☐	☐	_____
5. If the side rails are in use, lower the side rail on the working side of the bed. The side rail on the opposite side of the bed should remain up. Lower the head of the bed so that the bed is flat (as tolerated).	☐	☐	_____
6. Ask the person to lie on his side, facing away from you, in Sims' position. Help the person into this position, if necessary.	☐	☐	_____
7. Fanfold the top linens to below the person's buttocks. Adjust the person's hospital gown or pajama bottoms as necessary to expose the person's buttocks.	☐	☐	_____
8. Put on the gloves.	☐	☐	_____
9. With one hand, raise the person's upper buttock to expose the anus. Suggest that the person take a deep breath and slowly exhale as the thermometer is inserted. Using your other hand, gently and carefully insert the lubricated end of the thermometer into the person's rectum (not more than 1 inch for adults, or ½ inch for children). Never force the thermometer	☐	☐	_____

into the rectum. If you are unable to insert the thermometer, stop and call the nurse.

10. Hold the thermometer in place for the specified amount of time:

   a. **Glass thermometer:** 3 to 5 minutes (or follow facility policy) ☐ ☐ _____

   b. **Electronic thermometer:** until the instrument blinks or beeps (usually just a few seconds) ☐ ☐ _____

11. Remove the thermometer from the person's rectum. Wipe the person's anal area with a tissue to remove the lubricant, and adjust the person's hospital gown or pajama bottoms as necessary to cover the buttocks. ☐ ☐ _____

12. Read the temperature measurement.

   a. **Glass thermometer:** Using a tissue, remove the thermometer sheath from the glass thermometer, being careful not to touch the bulb end of the thermometer. Dispose of the tissue and the thermometer sheath in a facility-approved waste container. Hold the thermometer horizontally by the stem at eye level while facing a light source. Rotate the thermometer until you can see the level of the indicator material. Read the temperature. ☐ ☐ _____

   b. **Electronic thermometer:** Read the temperature on the electronic thermometer's display screen. Remove the probe sheath from the probe by pushing the button on the top of the probe. Direct the probe sheath into a facility-approved waste container. ☐ ☐ _____

13. Remove your gloves and dispose of them according to facility policy. Wash your hands. ☐ ☐ _____

14. Note the person's name, the time, the temperature, and the method on your notepad (or record the temperature and the method on the person's medical record if it is kept at the bedside). Place an "R" (or the notation designated by your facility) next to the measurement to indicate that the measurement was taken rectally. Report an abnormal temperature to the nurse immediately. ☐ ☐ _____

15. Help the person back into a comfortable position, straighten the bottom linens, and draw the top linens over the person. Raise the head of the bed, as the person requests. ☐ ☐ _____

16. Make sure that the bed is lowered to its lowest position and that the wheels are locked. If the side rails are in use, return the side rails to the raised position. ☐ ☐ _____

17. Prepare the thermometer for its next use.

   a. **Glass thermometer:** Shake down the glass thermometer, clean it according to facility policy, and return it to its disinfectant-filled case. ☐ ☐ _____

b. **Electronic thermometer:** Replace the probe into the electronic thermometer. (Always read the temperature before placing the probe in the instrument because this action clears the display screen.) Turn the instrument off if it does not automatically turn itself off. Place the thermometer in its charger.

☐ ☐ _____

Finishing Up

18. Complete the "Finishing Up" steps.

☐ ☐ _____

PROCEDURE 17-3
Measuring an Axillary Temperature (Glass or Electronic Thermometer)

Getting Ready	S	U	COMMENTS
1. Complete the "Getting Ready" steps.	☐	☐	_____

Procedure

2. Ask the person if she has bathed or applied deodorant or antiperspirant within the last 15 minutes. If so, wait 15 to 30 minutes before proceeding (or follow facility policy). ☐ ☐ _____

3. Prepare the thermometer.

   a. **Glass thermometer:** Run cool water over the thermometer to rinse away the disinfectant. Dry the thermometer with a paper towel and inspect it for cracks or chips. Carefully shake down the glass thermometer so that the indicator material is below the 94° mark (if using a Fahrenheit thermometer) or the 34° mark (if using a Celsius thermometer). Cover the end of the glass thermometer with the thermometer sheath. ☐ ☐ _____

   b. **Electronic thermometer:** Cover the electronic probe with the probe sheath. Turn the thermometer on and wait until the "ready" sign appears on the display screen. ☐ ☐ _____

4. Assist the person with removing her arm from the sleeve of her hospital gown or pajama top. ☐ ☐ _____

5. Pat the axilla (underarm area) gently with a paper towel. ☐ ☐ _____

6. Ask the person to lift her arm slightly. Position the tip of the thermometer in the center of the axilla and ask the person to hold the thermometer in place by holding her arm close to the body (or by grasping the arm with the opposite hand).

7. Leave the thermometer in place for the specified amount of time:

   a. **Glass thermometer:** 10 minutes (or follow facility policy) ☐ ☐ _____

   b. **Electronic thermometer:** until the instrument blinks or beeps (usually just a few seconds) ☐ ☐ _____

8. Ask the person to lift her arm slightly. Remove the thermometer. ☐ ☐ _____

9. Read the temperature measurement.

   a. **Glass thermometer:** Using a tissue, remove the thermometer sheath from the glass thermometer, being careful not to touch the bulb end of the thermometer. Dispose of the tissue and the thermometer sheath in a facility-approved waste ☐ ☐ _____

container. Hold the thermometer horizontally by the stem at eye level while facing a light source. Rotate the thermometer until you can see the level of the indicator material. Read the temperature.

b. **Electronic thermometer:** Read the temperature on the electronic thermometer's display screen. Remove the probe sheath from the probe by pushing the button on the top of the probe. Direct the probe sheath into a facility-approved waste container. ☐ ☐ _____

10. Note the person's name, the time, the temperature, and the method on your notepad (or record the temperature and the method on the person's medical record, if it is kept at the bedside). Place an "A" (or the notation designated by your facility) next to the measurement to indicate that the measurement was taken in the axilla. Report an abnormal temperature to the nurse immediately. ☐ ☐ _____

11. Help the person back into her hospital gown or pajama top. ☐ ☐ _____

12. Prepare the thermometer for its next use:

a. **Glass thermometer:** Shake down the glass thermometer, clean it according to facility policy, and return it to its disinfectant-filled case. ☐ ☐ _____

b. **Electronic thermometer:** Replace the probe into the electronic thermometer. (Always read the temperature before placing the probe in the instrument because this action clears the display screen.) Turn the instrument off, if it does not automatically turn itself off. Place the thermometer in its charger. ☐ ☐ _____

Finishing Up

13. Complete the "Finishing Up" steps. ☐ ☐ _____

PROCEDURE 17-4
Measuring a Tympanic Temperature (Tympanic Thermometer)

Getting Ready	S	U	COMMENTS
1. Complete the "Getting Ready" steps.	☐	☐	_____

Procedure

	S	U	COMMENTS
2. If the person wears a hearing aid, remove it carefully and wait 2 minutes before taking the person's temperature.	☐	☐	_____
3. Inspect the ear canal for excessive cerumen (ear wax). If you see excessive wax build-up in the ear canal, gently wipe the ear canal with a warm, moist washcloth.	☐	☐	_____
4. Cover the cone-shaped end of the thermometer with the probe sheath. Turn the thermometer on and wait until the "ready" sign appears on the display screen.	☐	☐	_____
5. Stand slightly to the front of, and facing, the person. To straighten the ear canal (which will ease insertion of the thermometer), grasp the top portion of the person's ear and gently pull:			
a. Up and back (in an adult)	☐	☐	_____
b. Straight back (in a child)	☐	☐	_____
6. Insert the covered probe into the person's ear canal, pointing the probe down and toward the front of the ear canal (pretend that you are aiming for the person's nose). This will seal off the ear canal by seating the probe properly, leading to a more accurate temperature reading.	☐	☐	_____
7. To take the temperature, press the button on the instrument. Keep the button depressed and the probe in place until the instrument blinks or beeps (usually 1 second).	☐	☐	_____
8. Remove the probe and read the temperature on the display screen.	☐	☐	_____
9. Remove the probe sheath from the probe by pushing the button on the side of the instrument. Direct the probe sheath into a facility-approved waste container.	☐	☐	_____
10. Note the person's name, the time, the temperature, and the method on your notepad (or record the temperature and method on the person's medical record if it is kept at the bedside). Place a "T" (or the notation designated by your facility) next to the measurement to indicate that the measurement was taken in the ear (i.e., using a tympanic thermometer). Report an abnormal temperature to the nurse immediately.	☐	☐	_____

11. If your facility requires a tympanic temperature to be taken in both ears, repeat the procedure, using a clean probe cover for the other ear.

☐ ☐ _____

12. Turn the instrument off if it does not automatically turn itself off. Place the thermometer in its charger.

☐ ☐ _____

Finishing Up

13. Complete the "Finishing Up" steps.

☐ ☐ _____

PROCEDURE 17-5
Taking a Radial Pulse

Getting Ready	S	U	COMMENTS

1. Complete the "Getting Ready" steps. ☐ ☐ _____

Procedure

2. Rest the person's arm on the over-bed table or on the bed. Locate the radial pulse in the person's wrist using your middle two or three fingers. (TIP: The radial pulse will be on the person's "thumb" side.) ☐ ☐ _____

3. Note the strength and regularity of the pulse. Look at your watch and wait until the second hand gets to the "12" or "6." When the second hand reaches the "12" or the "6," begin counting the pulse.

   a. If the pulse rhythm is regular, count the number of pulses that occur in 30 seconds and multiply the result by 2 to arrive at the pulse rate. ☐ ☐ _____

   b. If the pulse rhythm is irregular, count the number of pulses that occur in 60 seconds. Counting each pulse that occurs over the course of 1 full minute is the only way to obtain a truly accurate pulse rate when the pulse is irregular. ☐ ☐ _____

4. Note the person's name; the time; and the pulse rate, rhythm, and amplitude on your notepad (or record the pulse rate, rhythm, and amplitude on the person's medical record if it is kept at the bedside). Report an abnormal pulse rate, rhythm, or amplitude to the nurse immediately. ☐ ☐ _____

Finishing Up

5. Complete the "Finishing Up" steps. ☐ ☐ _____

PROCEDURE 17-6
Taking an Apical Pulse

	S	U	COMMENTS

Getting Ready

1. Complete the "Getting Ready" steps. ☐ ☐ _____

Procedure

2. Help the person to a sitting position by raising the head of the bed. ☐ ☐ _____

3. Using alcohol wipes, clean the earpieces, the diaphragm, and the bell of the stethoscope. Place the earpieces in your ears. ☐ ☐ _____

4. Place the diaphragm (or the bell, if the person is a child or infant) of the stethoscope under the person's clothing, on the apical pulse site (located approximately 2 inches below the person's left nipple). The diaphragm or bell must be placed directly on the person's skin because clothing will distort the sound. ☐ ☐ _____

5. Using two fingers, hold the diaphragm or bell firmly against the person's chest. Look at your watch and wait until the second hand gets to the "12" or "6." When the second hand reaches the "12" or the "6," begin counting the heartbeat. ☐ ☐ _____

6. Count the number of heartbeats that occur in 60 seconds. Each time the heart beats, you will hear two sounds, best described as a "lubb" and a "dupp." Both sounds make up one beat of the heart and should be counted as such. ☐ ☐ _____

7. After 60 seconds, remove the diaphragm of the stethoscope from the person's chest. Adjust the person's clothing as necessary and help the person back into a comfortable position. Lower the head of the bed, as the person requests. ☐ ☐ _____

8. Note the person's name; the time; the pulse rate, rhythm, and amplitude; and the method on your notepad (or record the pulse rate, rhythm, and amplitude and the method on the person's medical record if it is kept at the bedside). Place an "a" (or the notation designated by your facility) next to the measurement to indicate that the measurement was taken apically. Report an abnormal pulse to the nurse immediately. ☐ ☐ _____

9. Using alcohol wipes, clean the earpieces, the diaphragm, and the bell of the stethoscope. ☐ ☐ _____

Finishing Up

10. Complete the "Finishing Up" steps. ☐ ☐ _____

PROCEDURE 17-7
Counting Respirations

	S	U	COMMENTS

Getting Ready

1. Complete the "Getting Ready" steps.   ☐ ☐ _____

Procedure

2. Look at your watch and wait until the second hand gets to the "12" or "6." When the second hand reaches the "12" or the "6," look at the person's chest (or place your hand near the person's collarbone or on his side) and begin counting each rise and fall of the chest as one breath.

   a. If the respiratory rhythm is regular, count the number of breaths that occur in 30 seconds and multiply the result by 2 to arrive at the respiratory rate.   ☐ ☐ _____

   b. If the respiratory rhythm is irregular, count the number of breaths that occur in 60 seconds. Counting each respiration that occurs over the course of 1 full minute is the only way to obtain a truly accurate respiratory rate when the person's breathing is irregular.   ☐ ☐ _____

3. Note the person's name, the time, and the respiratory rate on your notepad (or record the respiratory rate on the person's medical record if it is kept at the bedside). Report abnormal respirations to the nurse immediately.   ☐ ☐ _____

Finishing Up

4. Complete the "Finishing Up" steps.   ☐ ☐ _____

PROCEDURE 17-8
Measuring Blood Pressure

Getting Ready	S	U	COMMENTS
1. Complete the "Getting Ready" steps.	☐	☐	_____

Procedure

	S	U	COMMENTS
2. Assist the person into a sitting or lying position. Position the person's arm so that the forearm is level with the heart and the palm of the hand is facing upward. Assist the person with rolling up her sleeve so that the upper arm is exposed.	☐	☐	_____
3. Using alcohol wipes, clean the earpieces, the diaphragm, and the bell of the stethoscope.	☐	☐	_____
4. Stand no more than 3 feet away from the manometer. If it is not mounted on the wall, stand a mercury manometer upright on a flat surface, at eye level. Lay an aneroid manometer on a flat surface directly in front of you or leave it attached to the blood pressure cuff.	☐	☐	_____
5. Squeeze the cuff to empty it of any remaining air. Turn the valve on the bulb clockwise to close it; this will cause the cuff to inflate when you pump the bulb.	☐	☐	_____
6. Locate the person's brachial artery in the antecubital space by placing your fingers at the inner aspect of the elbow.	☐	☐	_____
7. Place the arrow mark on the cuff over the brachial artery. Wrap the cuff around the person's upper arm so that the bottom of the cuff is at least 1 inch above the person's elbow. The cuff must be even and snug.	☐	☐	_____
8. Place the stethoscope earpieces in your ears.	☐	☐	_____
9. Pump the bulb until the pressure in the cuff is 30 mm Hg higher than the systolic pressure. There are two ways to do this:			
Method "A." Hold the bulb in one hand and position the diaphragm of the stethoscope over the brachial artery with the other hand. Inflate the cuff until you hear the pulse stop and then inflate the cuff 30 mm Hg more.	☐	☐	_____
Method "B." Hold the bulb in one hand and feel for the person's radial pulse (in her wrist) with the other hand. Inflate the cuff until you are no longer able to feel the radial pulse and then inflate the cuff 30 mm Hg more.	☐	☐	_____
10. Position the diaphragm of the stethoscope over the brachial artery (or continue to hold it there if you used method "A" to inflate the cuff).	☐	☐	_____

11. Turn the valve on the bulb slightly counterclockwise to allow air to escape from the cuff slowly.

☐ ☐ _____

12. Note the reading on the manometer where the first sound of the brachial pulse is heard. This is the systolic reading.

☐ ☐ _____

13. Continue to deflate the cuff. Note the reading on the manometer where the last sound of the brachial pulse is heard. This is the diastolic reading.

☐ ☐ _____

14. Deflate the cuff completely and remove it from the person's arm. Remove the stethoscope from your ears.

☐ ☐ _____

15. Note the person's name, the time, and the blood pressure on your notepad (or record the blood pressure on the person's medical record if it is kept at the bedside). Report an abnormal blood pressure to the nurse immediately.

☐ ☐ _____

16. Return the sphygmomanometer to its case or wall holder.

☐ ☐ _____

17. Using alcohol wipes, clean the earpieces, the diaphragm, and the bell of the stethoscope.

☐ ☐ _____

Finishing Up

18. Complete the "Finishing Up" steps.

☐ ☐ _____

PROCEDURE 17-9
Measuring Height and Weight Using an Upright Scale

	S	U	COMMENTS

Getting Ready

1. Complete the "Getting Ready" steps. ☐ ☐ _____

Procedure

2. Ask the person to urinate. If necessary, assist the person to the bathroom or offer the bedpan or urinal. ☐ ☐ _____

3. Move the weights all the way to the left of the balance bar. ☐ ☐ _____

4. Help the person onto the scale platform so that she is facing the balance bar. Once the person is on the scale platform, do not allow her to hold on to you or to the scale. ☐ ☐ _____

5. Move the large weight on the lower scale bar to the right to the weight closest to the person's prior weight. For example, if the person weighed 155 pounds the last time you weighed her, you would move the large weight to the "150" mark. ☐ ☐ _____

6. Move the small weight on the upper scale bar to the right until the balance pointer is centered between the two scale bars. ☐ ☐ _____

7. Read the numbers on the upper and the lower scale bars where each weight has settled and add these two numbers together. This is the person's weight. ☐ ☐ _____

8. Have the person carefully turn around to face away from the scale bar. Slide the height scale up so that you can pull out the height rod, which extends from the top of the height scale. Be careful not to hit the person in the head with the height rod. ☐ ☐ _____

9. Slide the height rod down so that it lightly touches the top of the person's head. Read the number at the point where the height rod meets the height scale. This is the person's height. ☐ ☐ _____

10. Hold the height rod in your hand, and help the person step down from the scale. ☐ ☐ _____

11. Assist the person back to her room. ☐ ☐ _____

12. Note the person's name, the time, and the weight and height on your notepad (or record the weight and height on the person's medical record if it is kept at the bedside). Report a change in the person's weight to the nurse. ☐ ☐ _____

Finishing Up

13. Complete the "Finishing Up" steps. ☐ ☐ _____

PROCEDURE 17-10
Measuring Weight Using a Chair Scale

	S	U	COMMENTS

Getting Ready

1. Complete the "Getting Ready" steps. □ □ _____

Procedure

2. Ask the person to urinate. If necessary, assist the person to the bathroom or offer the bedpan or urinal. □ □ _____

3. Assist or wheel the person to the scale, using a transfer belt, a wheelchair, or both. □ □ _____

4. Reset the scale to "0" by turning it on. □ □ _____

5. Help the person onto the scale.

  a. If a regular chair scale is being used, help the person to sit in the chair on the scale. Make sure the person is seated properly, with her buttocks against the back of the chair and feet on the footrests. □ □ _____

  b. If a wheelchair scale is being used, roll the occupied wheelchair onto the platform and lock the wheels. □ □ _____

6. Read the weight on the display screen. If a wheelchair scale is being used, you must subtract the weight of the unoccupied wheelchair from this figure to determine the person's weight. □ □ _____

7. Help the person off of the scale.

  a. If a regular chair scale is being used, assist the person out of the chair and back into a wheelchair if one was used for the transfer. □ □ _____

  b. If a wheelchair scale is being used, unlock the wheels and roll the wheelchair off the platform. □ □ _____

8. Assist the person back to her room. □ □ _____

9. Note the person's name, the time, and the weight on your notepad (or record the weight on the person's medical record if it is kept at the bedside). Report a change in the person's weight to the nurse. □ □ _____

Finishing Up

10. Complete the "Finishing Up" steps. □ □ _____

CHAPTER 18 PROCEDURE CHECKLISTS

PROCEDURE 18-1
Brushing and Flossing the Teeth

	S	U	COMMENTS

Getting Ready

1. Complete the "Getting Ready" steps. ☐ ☐ _____

Procedure

2. Cover the over-bed table with paper towels. Place the oral care supplies on the over-bed table. Fill a paper cup with water. ☐ ☐ _____

3. Make sure that the bed is positioned at a comfortable working height (to promote good body mechanics) and that the wheels are locked. ☐ ☐ _____

4. If the side rails are in use, lower the side rail on the working side of the bed. The side rail on the opposite side of the bed should remain up. ☐ ☐ _____

5. Raise the head of the bed as tolerated. Place a towel under the person's chin. ☐ ☐ _____

6. Put on the gloves. ☐ ☐ _____

7. Wet the toothbrush. Put a small amount of toothpaste on the toothbrush. ☐ ☐ _____

8. Brush the person's teeth as follows:

   a. Position the toothbrush at a 45° angle to the gums, against the outer surface of the top teeth. Starting at the back of the mouth, brush the outer surface of each tooth using a gentle circular motion. Repeat for the lower teeth. Allow the person to spit toothpaste into the emesis basin as necessary. ☐ ☐ _____

   b. Position the toothbrush at a 45° angle to the gums, against the inner surface of the top teeth. Starting at the back of the mouth, brush the inner surface of each tooth using a gentle circular motion. Repeat for the lower teeth. ☐ ☐ _____

   c. Brush the chewing surfaces of the upper and lower teeth using a gentle circular motion. ☐ ☐ _____

   d. Brush the tongue. ☐ ☐ _____

9. Offer the person the cup of water (and a straw, if desired) and ask her to rinse her mouth completely. Hold the emesis basin underneath the person's chin so that she can spit the water into the basin. ☐ ☐ _____

10. Place the emesis basin on the over-bed table and dry the person's mouth and chin thoroughly using a towel. ☐ ☐ _____

11. Cut a piece of dental floss measuring about 18 inches. Wrap the dental floss around the middle finger of each hand. Hold the dental floss between your thumb and index finger on each hand and stretch it tight.

☐ ☐ _____

12. Insert a segment of dental floss between two teeth, starting with the back upper teeth. Move the floss up and down gently, and then remove the dental floss from the person's mouth. Advance the floss a bit by releasing it from one middle finger and wrapping it around the other, and move on to the next two teeth. Use a new strand of dental floss as necessary. Offer the person the glass of water (and the straw, if desired) to rinse as necessary. Floss all of the person's teeth.

☐ ☐ _____

13. Offer the person the cup of water (and the straw, if desired) and ask her to rinse her mouth completely. Hold the emesis basin underneath the person's chin so that she can spit the water into the basin.

☐ ☐ _____

14. Place the emesis basin on the over-bed table and dry the person's mouth and chin thoroughly using a towel.

☐ ☐ _____

15. Pour a small amount of mouthwash (approximately ¼ cup) into another paper cup and help the person to rinse, as the person requests.

☐ ☐ _____

16. Apply lip lubricant to the lips, as the person requests.

☐ ☐ _____

17. If the side rails are in use, return the side rails to the raised position. Lower the head of the bed as the person requests. Make sure that the bed is lowered to its lowest position and that the wheels are locked.

☐ ☐ _____

18. Gather the soiled linens and place them in the linen hamper or linen bag. Dispose of disposable items in a facility-approved waste container. Clean equipment and return it to the storage area.

☐ ☐ _____

19. Remove your gloves and dispose of them in a facility-approved waste container.

☐ ☐ _____

Finishing Up

20. Complete the "Finishing Up" steps.

☐ ☐ _____

PROCEDURE 18-2
Providing Oral Care for a Person With Dentures

Getting Ready

	S	U	COMMENTS
1. Complete the "Getting Ready" steps.	☐	☐	_____

Procedure

	S	U	COMMENTS
2. Cover the over-bed table with paper towels. Place the oral care supplies on the over-bed table. Fill a paper cup with water.	☐	☐	_____
3. Make sure that the bed is positioned at a comfortable working height (to promote good body mechanics) and that the wheels are locked. Raise the head of the bed as tolerated. Place a towel under the person's chin.	☐	☐	_____
4. Put on the gloves.	☐	☐	_____
5. Ask the person to remove his dentures and place them in the emesis basin. If the person needs assistance with removing his dentures:			
a. Ask the person to open his mouth.	☐	☐	_____
b. Holding a gauze square between your thumb and index finger, grasp the upper denture, moving it up and down slightly to break the seal. Ease the denture down, forward, and out of the mouth. Place the denture in the emesis basin.	☐	☐	_____
c. Holding a gauze square between your thumb and index finger, grasp the lower denture. Turn the denture slightly, lifting it out of the mouth. Place the denture in the emesis basin.	☐	☐	_____
6. Take the emesis basin, the washcloth, the denture cup, the denture brush or toothbrush, and the denture cleaner or toothpaste to the sink. Line the sink with the washcloth to provide extra cushioning. Fill the sink partially with lukewarm water. Do not place the dentures in the sink.	☐	☐	_____
7. Wet the denture brush or the toothbrush. Put a small amount of toothpaste or denture cleaner on the denture brush or toothbrush. Working with one denture at a time, hold the denture in the palm of your hand and brush it on all surfaces until it is clean. Rinse the denture thoroughly under lukewarm running water and place it in the denture cup. Repeat with the other denture.	☐	☐	_____
8. If the dentures are to be stored, fill the denture cup with lukewarm water, a mixture of one part mouthwash to one part lukewarm water, or a denture solution so that the dentures are covered. Put the lid on the denture cup. Return the denture cup to the person's bedside table, making sure that it is within easy reach.	☐	☐	_____

9. If the dentures are to be reinserted in the person's mouth, take the emesis basin, the denture cup, and the toothbrush to the over-bed table. If the side rails are in use, lower the side rail on the working side of the bed. The side rail on the opposite side of the bed should remain up.

   a. Offer the person the cup of water (and a straw, if desired) and ask him to rinse his mouth completely. Some people may wish to use mouthwash instead of water. Hold the emesis basin underneath the person's chin so that he can spit the water or mouthwash into the basin.

   b. Place the emesis basin on the over-bed table and dry the person's mouth and chin thoroughly using a face towel.

   c. Gently clean the person's gums and tongue and the insides of the cheeks with the toothbrush or a foam-tipped applicator moistened with water or mouthwash. Use fresh applicators as needed.

   d. Ask the person to insert his dentures. If the person needs assistance with inserting his dentures:

     ■ Ask the person to open his mouth.

     ■ Gently lift the person's upper lip up. Grasp the upper denture between your thumb and index finger and insert it in the person's mouth. Press gently on the denture to be sure that it is seated properly.

     ■ Gently pull the person's lower lip down. Grasp the lower denture between your thumb and index finger and insert it in the person's mouth.

   e. Return the denture cup to the person's bedside table, making sure that it is within easy reach.

10. Dry the person's mouth and chin thoroughly using a towel. Apply lip lubricant to the lips, as the person requests.

11. Reposition the person comfortably and lower the head of the bed if necessary. If the side rails are in use, return the side rails to the raised position. Make sure that the bed is lowered to its lowest position and that the wheels are locked.

12. Gather the soiled linens and place them in the linen hamper or linen bag. Dispose of disposable items in a facility-approved waste container. Clean equipment and return it to the storage area.

13. Remove your gloves and dispose of them in a facility-approved waste container.

Finishing Up

14. Complete the "Finishing Up" steps.

PROCEDURE 18-3
Providing Oral Care for an Unconscious Person

	S	U	COMMENTS
Getting Ready			
1. Complete the "Getting Ready" steps.	☐	☐	_____

Procedure

	S	U	COMMENTS
2. Cover the over-bed table with paper towels. Place the oral care supplies on the over-bed table. Fill the paper cup with water.	☐	☐	_____
3. Make sure that the bed is positioned at a comfortable working height (to promote good body mechanics) and that the wheels are locked. If the side rails are in use, lower the side rail on the working side of the bed. The side rail on the opposite side of the bed should remain up.	☐	☐	_____
4. Raise the head of the bed as tolerated. Turn the person's head to the side facing you. If it is difficult to keep the person's head turned to the side, roll the person onto her side.	☐	☐	_____
5. If the person's condition permits, gently lift the person's head and place a towel on the pillow. Place the emesis basin on the towel, level with the person's chin.	☐	☐	_____
6. Put on the gloves.	☐	☐	_____
7. Open the person's mouth using the padded tongue blade. Be gentle; do not force the mouth open. Insert the tongue blade between the upper and lower teeth at the back of the mouth to hold the person's mouth open.	☐	☐	_____
8. Clean the inside of the mouth:			
a. If the person has natural teeth, they should be gently brushed as described in Procedure 18-1.	☐	☐	_____
b. If the person is edentulous, gently clean the person's gums and tongue and the insides of the cheeks with the toothbrush or a foam-tipped applicator moistened with water, saline, or mouthwash. Use fresh applicators as needed.	☐	☐	_____
9. Dry the person's mouth and chin thoroughly using a towel. Apply lip lubricant to the lips. Reposition the person comfortably.	☐	☐	_____
10. If the side rails are in use, return the side rails to the raised position. Lower the head of the bed. Make sure that the bed is lowered to its lowest position and that the wheels are locked.	☐	☐	_____
11. Gather the soiled linens and place them in the linen hamper or linen bag. Dispose of disposable items in a facility-approved waste container. Clean equipment and return it to the storage area.	☐	☐	_____

12. Remove your gloves and dispose of them in a facility-approved waste container.

☐ ☐ _____

Finishing Up

13. Complete the "Finishing Up" steps.

☐ ☐ _____

PROCEDURE 18-4
Providing Female Perineal Care

Getting Ready	S	U	COMMENTS
1. Complete the "Getting Ready" steps.	☐	☐	_____

Procedure

	S	U	COMMENTS
2. Cover the over-bed table with paper towels. Place the wash basin, toiletries, clean clothing, and clean linens on the over-bed table.	☐	☐	_____
3. Make sure that the bed is positioned at a comfortable working height (to promote good body mechanics) and that the wheels are locked.	☐	☐	_____
4. Put on the gloves.	☐	☐	_____
5. Because bathing often stimulates the urge to urinate, offer the bedpan. If the person uses the bedpan, empty and clean it before proceeding with the perineal care. Remove your gloves and dispose of them in a facility-approved waste container. Wash your hands and put on a clean pair of gloves.	☐	☐	_____
6. Lower the head of the bed to a flat position (as tolerated).	☐	☐	_____
7. Fill the wash basin with warm water [110°F (43.3°C) to 115°F (46.1°C) on the bath thermometer]. Place the basin on the over-bed table.	☐	☐	_____
8. If the side rails are in use, lower the side rail on the working side. The side rail on the opposite side of the bed should remain up.	☐	☐	_____
9. Spread the bath blanket over the top linens (and the person). If the person is able, have her hold the bath blanket. If not, tuck the corners under the person's shoulders. Fanfold the top linens to the foot of the bed.	☐	☐	_____
10. Assist the person with undressing.	☐	☐	_____
11. Ask the person to open her legs and bend her knees, if possible. If she is not able to bend her knees, help her spread her legs as much as possible.	☐	☐	_____
12. Position the bath blanket over the person so that one corner can be wrapped under and around each leg.	☐	☐	_____
13. Position the bed protector under the person's buttocks to keep the bed linens dry.	☐	☐	_____
14. Lift the corner of the bath blanket that is between the person's legs upward, exposing only the perineal area.	☐	☐	_____
15. Form a mitt around your hand with one of the washcloths. Wet the mitt with warm, clean water and apply soap.	☐	☐	_____

16. Using the other hand, separate the labia. Clean the vulva by placing your washcloth-covered hand at the top of the vulva and stroking downward to the anus. Use a different part of the washcloth for each stroke. Repeat until the area is clean. ☐ ☐ _____

17. Rinse the vulva and perineum thoroughly:

Method "A": Form a mitt around your hand with a clean, wet washcloth. Using the other hand, separate the labia. Rinse the vulva by placing your washcloth-covered hand at the top of the vulva and stroking downward to the anus. Use a different part of the washcloth for each stroke. Repeat until the area is free of soap. ☐ ☐ _____

Method "B": Hold a clean washcloth saturated with clean, warm water over the vulva. Squeeze the water from the washcloth onto the vulva and allow it to run over the vulva and perineum. Repeat until the area is free of soap. ☐ ☐ _____

18. Dry the perineal area thoroughly using a towel. ☐ ☐ _____

19. Turn the person onto her side so that she is facing away from you. Help the person toward the working side of the bed so that her buttocks are within easy reach. Adjust the bath blanket to keep the person covered. ☐ ☐ _____

20. Form a mitt around your hand with one of the washcloths. Wet the mitt with warm, clean water and apply soap. ☐ ☐ _____

21. Using the other hand, separate the buttocks. Place your washcloth-covered hand at the front of the body and stroke toward the back. First clean one side, then the other side, and finally the middle, using a different part of the washcloth each time, until the anal area is clean. ☐ ☐ _____

22. Rinse and dry the anal area thoroughly. Remove the bed protector from underneath the person. ☐ ☐ _____

23. Remove your gloves and dispose of them in a facility-approved waste container. Put on a clean pair of gloves. ☐ ☐ _____

24. Assist the person into the supine position. Reposition the pillow under her head. Remove the bath blanket and help the person into the clean clothing. ☐ ☐ _____

25. If the bedding is wet or soiled, change the bed linens. ☐ ☐ _____

26. If the side rails are in use, return the side rail to the raised position. Raise the head of the bed as the person requests. Make sure that the bed is lowered to its lowest position and that the wheels are locked. ☐ ☐ _____

27. Gather the soiled linens and place them in the linen hamper or linen bag. Dispose of disposable items in a facility-approved waste container. Clean equipment and return it to the storage area. ☐ ☐ _____

28. Remove your gloves and dispose of them in a facility-approved waste container.   ☐ ☐ _____

Finishing Up

29. Complete the "Finishing Up" steps.   ☐ ☐ _____

PROCEDURE 18-5
Providing Male Perineal Care

Getting Ready	S	U	COMMENTS
1. Complete the "Getting Ready" steps.	☐	☐	_____

Procedure

	S	U	COMMENTS
2. Cover the over-bed table with paper towels. Place the wash basin, toiletries, clean clothing, and clean linens on the over-bed table.	☐	☐	_____
3. Make sure that the bed is positioned at a comfortable working height (to promote good body mechanics) and that the wheels are locked.	☐	☐	_____
4. Put on the gloves.	☐	☐	_____
5. Because bathing often stimulates the urge to urinate, offer the bedpan or urinal. If the person uses the bedpan or urinal, empty and clean it before proceeding with the perineal care. Remove your gloves and dispose of them in a facility-approved waste container. Wash your hands and put on a clean pair of gloves.	☐	☐	_____
6. Lower the head of the bed to a flat position (as tolerated).	☐	☐	_____
7. Fill the wash basin with warm water [110°F (43.3°C) to 115°F (46.1°C) on the bath thermometer]. Place the basin on the over-bed table.	☐	☐	_____
8. If the side rails are in use, lower the side rail on the working side. The side rail on the opposite side of the bed should remain up.	☐	☐	_____
9. Spread the bath blanket over the top linens (and the person). If the person is able, have him hold the bath blanket. If not, tuck the corners under the person's shoulders. Fanfold the top linens to the foot of the bed.	☐	☐	_____
10. Assist the person with undressing.	☐	☐	_____
11. Ask the person to open his legs and bend his knees, if possible. If he is not able to bend his knees, help him spread his legs as much as possible.	☐	☐	_____
12. Position the bath blanket over the person so that one corner can be wrapped under and around each leg.	☐	☐	_____
13. Position the bed protector under the person's buttocks to keep the bed linens dry.	☐	☐	_____
14. Lift the corner of the bath blanket that is between the person's legs upward, exposing only the perineal area.	☐	☐	_____
15. Form a mitt around your hand with one of the washcloths. Wet the mitt with warm, clean water and apply soap.	☐	☐	_____

16. Using the other hand, hold the penis slightly away from the body.

   a. If the person is circumcised: Place your washcloth-covered hand at the tip of the penis and wash in a circular motion, downward to the base of the penis. Repeat, using a different part of the washcloth each time, until the area is clean. Rinse and dry the tip and the shaft of the penis thoroughly:

   Method "A": Form a mitt around your hand with a clean, wet washcloth. Using the other hand, hold the penis slightly away from the body. Place your washcloth-covered hand at the tip of the penis and wipe in a circular motion, downward to the base of the penis. Repeat, using a different part of the washcloth each time, until the area is rinsed. Dry the penis thoroughly.

   Method "B": Hold a clean washcloth saturated with clean, warm water over the area. Squeeze the water from the washcloth onto the area. Dry the penis thoroughly.

   b. If the person is uncircumcised: Retract the foreskin by gently pushing the skin toward the base of the penis. Place your washcloth-covered hand at the tip of the penis and wash in a circular motion, downward to the base of the penis. Repeat using a different part of the washcloth each time until the area is clean. Rinse and dry the tip and shaft of the penis thoroughly before gently pulling the foreskin back into its normal position.

17. Form a mitt around your hand with one of the washcloths. Wet the mitt with warm, clean water and apply soap. Wash the scrotum and perineum. Rinse and dry the scrotum and perineum thoroughly.

18. Turn the person onto his side so that he is facing away from you. Help the person toward the working side of the bed so that his buttocks are within easy reach. Adjust the bath blanket to keep the person covered.

19. Form a mitt around your hand with one of the washcloths. Wet the mitt with warm, clean water and apply soap.

20. Using the other hand, separate the buttocks. Place your washcloth-covered hand at the front of the body and stroke toward the back. First clean one side, then the other side, and finally the middle, using a different part of the washcloth each time, until the anal area is clean.

21. Rinse and dry the anal area thoroughly. Remove the bed protector from underneath the person.

22. Remove your gloves and dispose of them in a facility-approved waste container. Put on a clean pair of gloves.   ☐ ☐ _____

23. Assist the person into the supine position. Reposition the pillow under the person's head. Remove the bath blanket and help the person into the clean clothing.   ☐ ☐ _____

24. If the bedding is wet or soiled, change the bed linens.   ☐ ☐ _____

25. If the side rails are in use, return the side rail to the raised position. Make sure that the bed is lowered to its lowest position and that the wheels are locked.   ☐ ☐ _____

26. Gather the soiled linens and place them in the linen hamper or linen bag. Dispose of disposable items in a facility-approved waste container. Clean equipment and return it to the storage area.   ☐ ☐ _____

27. Remove your gloves and dispose of them in a facility-approved waste container.   ☐ ☐ _____

Finishing Up

28. Complete the "Finishing Up" steps.   ☐ ☐ _____

PROCEDURE 18-6
Assisting With a Tub Bath or Shower

Getting Ready	S	U	COMMENTS

1. Prepare the tub room. Place a nonskid mat on the floor of the tub or shower. If the person will be taking a tub bath, fill the tub halfway with warm water (105°F [43.3°C] to 115°F [46.1°C] on the bath thermometer). Obtain a shower chair if necessary and place it in the shower. Place a towel on the chair in the tub room where the person will sit while drying off. ☐ ☐ _____

2. Complete the "Getting Ready" steps. ☐ ☐ _____

Procedure

3. Ask the person if she needs to use the bathroom before bathing. ☐ ☐ _____

4. Assist the person to the tub room. ☐ ☐ _____

5. If the person will be taking a tub bath, check the temperature of the water and make sure the nonskid mat is secure. If the person will be taking a shower, turn on the water and adjust the temperature until the water is comfortable. ☐ ☐ _____

6. Assist the person with undressing. Assist the person into the bathtub or shower. ☐ ☐ _____

7. If the person is able to bathe herself, either partially or completely:

  a. Place bathing supplies within easy reach. ☐ ☐ _____

  b. Many facilities require you to remain in the room while the person bathes or showers. If facility policy permits you to leave the room, explain how to use the call-light control and ask the person to signal when bathing is complete or when she has done as much as she can on her own and needs help completing the bath. Stay nearby and check on the person every 5 minutes. The person should not remain in the bathtub or shower for longer than 20 minutes. Return when the person signals. Remember to knock before entering. ☐ ☐ _____

8. If the person is unable to bathe herself or requires assistance:

  a. Put on the gloves and form a mitt around your hand with one of the washcloths. ☐ ☐ _____

  b. If necessary, ask the person what parts of the body were not washed. Assist the person as needed with completing the bath. Wash the cleanest areas first and the dirtiest areas last: ☐ ☐ _____

- Eyes. Wet the mitt with warm, clean water. Ask the person to close her eyes. Place your washcloth-covered hand at the inner corner of the eye and stroke gently outward, toward the outer corner. Use a different part of the washcloth for each eye. □ □ _____

- Face, neck, and ears. Ask the person if you should use soap on the face. Rinse the washcloth and apply soap, if requested. Wash the face, neck, and ears, moving from the top of the head to the bottom (so that the nose and mouth are washed last). Rinse thoroughly. □ □ _____

- Arms and axillae (armpits). Rinse the washcloth and apply soap. Place your washcloth-covered hand at the shoulder and stroke downward, toward the hand, using long, firm strokes. Wash the hand. If necessary, assist the person with raising her arm so that you can wash the axilla. Repeat for the other arm and axilla. □ □ _____

- Chest and abdomen. Using long, firm strokes, wash the person's chest and abdomen. □ □ _____

- Legs and feet. Place your washcloth-covered hand at the top of the thigh and stroke downward, toward the foot, using long, firm strokes. Wash the foot. Repeat for the other leg. □ □ _____

- Back and buttocks: Wash the person's back and buttocks, moving from top to bottom and using long, firm strokes. □ □ _____

- Perineal area: Complete perineal care. □ □ _____

9. Make sure that soap is thoroughly rinsed from all parts of the body. □ □ _____

10. Remove your gloves and dispose of them in a facility-approved waste container. Put on a clean pair of gloves. □ □ _____

11. If the person is taking a tub bath, drain the water and carefully assist the person out of the tub and into the towel-covered chair. If the person is taking a shower, turn the water off and assist the person into the towel-covered chair. □ □ _____

12. Wrap a towel around the person. Using another bath towel, help the person to dry off, patting the skin dry. Take care to ensure that areas where "skin meets skin" are dried thoroughly (for example, in between the toes and underneath the breasts). □ □ _____

13. Help the person to apply lotion, powder, deodorant, antiperspirant, or other personal care products as the person requests. □ □ _____

14. Help the person into the clean clothing. If the person is wearing nightwear, help her into a robe. Help the person into her slippers. □ □ _____

15. Remove your gloves and dispose of them in a facility-approved waste container.

☐ ☐ _____

16. Assist the person back to her room.

☐ ☐ _____

Finishing Up

17. Complete the "Finishing Up" steps.

☐ ☐ _____

18. Gather the soiled linens and place them in the linen hamper or linen bag. Dispose of disposable items in a facility-approved waste container. Clean equipment and return it to the storage area.

☐ ☐ _____

19. Clean the tub room and shower chair (if used), if housekeeping is not responsible for this task at your facility.

☐ ☐ _____

PROCEDURE 18-7
Giving a Complete Bed Bath

	S	U	COMMENTS

Getting Ready

1. Complete the "Getting Ready" steps. ☐ ☐ _____

Procedure

2. Cover the over-bed table with paper towels. Place the wash basin, toiletries, clean clothing, and clean linens on the over-bed table. ☐ ☐ _____

3. Make sure that the bed is positioned at a comfortable working height (to promote good body mechanics) and that the wheels are locked. ☐ ☐ _____

4. Put on the gloves. ☐ ☐ _____

5. Because bathing often stimulates the urge to urinate, offer the bedpan or urinal. If the person uses the bedpan or urinal, empty and clean it before proceeding with the bath. Remove your gloves and dispose of them in a facility-approved waste container. Wash your hands and put on a clean pair of gloves. ☐ ☐

6. Assist the person with oral care. ☐ ☐ _____

7. Remove the bedspread and blanket from the bed. If they are to be reused, fold them and place them on a clean surface, such as the chair. ☐ ☐ _____

8. Spread the bath blanket over the top linens (and the person). If the person is able, have him hold the bath blanket. If not, tuck the corners under the person's shoulders. Fanfold the top linens to the foot of the bed. ☐ ☐ _____

9. Assist the person with undressing. ☐ ☐ _____

10. Lower the head of the bed so that the bed is flat (as tolerated). Position the pillow under the person's head. ☐ ☐ _____

11. Fill the wash basin with warm water [110°F (43.3°C) to 115°F (46.1°C) on the bath thermometer]. Place the basin on the over-bed table. ☐ ☐ _____

12. If the side rails are in use, lower the side rail on the working side of the bed. The side rail on the opposite side of the bed should remain up. ☐ ☐ _____

13. Place a towel over the person's chest to keep the bath blanket dry. ☐ ☐ _____

14. To keep the bath water from becoming soapy too quickly, you can use two washcloths—one with soap, for washing; and one without soap, for rinsing. Form a mitt around your hand with one of the washcloths. Wet the mitt with warm, clean water. Ask the person to close his eyes. Place your washcloth-covered hand at the inner corner of the eye and stroke gently outward, toward the outer corner. Use a different part of the washcloth for each eye. Using a towel, dry the person's eyes. ☐ ☐ _____

15. Ask the person if you should use soap on the face. Rinse the washcloth and apply soap, if requested. Wash the face, neck, and ears, moving from the top of the head to the bottom (so that the nose and mouth are washed last). Using the clean washcloth, rinse thoroughly, and pat the person's face, neck, and ears dry with a towel. ☐ ☐ _____

16. Place a bed protector under the person's far arm, to keep the linens dry. Form a mitt around your hand with the washcloth. Wet the mitt and apply soap. Place your washcloth-covered hand at the shoulder and stroke downward, toward the hand, using long, firm strokes. Wash the hand. If necessary, assist the person with raising his arm so that you can wash the axilla. Rinse thoroughly, and pat the person's arm, hand, and axilla dry with a towel. Remove the bed protector from underneath the person's arm. ☐ ☐ _____

17. Repeat for the other arm. ☐ ☐ _____

18. Place a towel horizontally across the person's chest. (The person is now covered with both a bath blanket and a towel.) With the towel in place, fold the bath blanket down to the person's waist. Wet the mitt and apply soap. Reach under the towel and wash the person's chest, using long, firm strokes. Using the clean washcloth, rinse thoroughly, and pat the person's chest dry with a towel. ☐ ☐ _____

19. With the towel still in place, fold the bath blanket down to the pubic area. Form a mitt around your hand with the washcloth. Wet the mitt and apply soap. Reach under the towel and wash the person's abdomen, using long, firm strokes. Rinse thoroughly and pat the person's abdomen dry with a towel. ☐ ☐ _____

20. Replace the bath blanket by unfolding it back over the towel and the person's body. Slide the towel out from underneath the bath blanket. ☐ ☐ _____

21. Change the water in the wash basin if it is cool or soapy. (If the side rails are in use, raise the side rails before leaving the bedside.) ☐ ☐ _____

22. Fold the bath blanket so that the far leg is completely exposed. Place a bed protector under the person's far leg to keep the linens dry. Wet the mitt and apply soap. Place your washcloth-covered hand at the top of the thigh and stroke downward, toward the foot, using long, firm strokes. Rinse thoroughly and pat the person's leg dry with a bath towel. ☐ ☐ _____

23. Put the wash basin on the bed protector and place the person's foot in the basin. Wash the entire foot, including between the toes, with the soapy washcloth. Rinse thoroughly and pat the person's foot dry with a towel. Be sure to dry between the toes. Remove the wash basin. Remove the bed protector from underneath the person's leg. ☐ ☐ _____

24. Repeat for the other leg and foot.   ☐ ☐ _____

25. Change the water in the wash basin. (If the side rails   ☐ ☐ _____
    are in use, raise the side rails before leaving the
    bedside.)

26. Turn the person onto his side so that he is facing   ☐ ☐ _____
    away from you. Help the person toward the working
    side of the bed so that his back is within easy reach.
    Adjust the bath blanket to keep the front of the
    person covered (exposing only the back and
    buttocks). Place a bed protector on the bed alongside
    the person's back to keep the linens dry.

27. Form a mitt around your hand with the washcloth.   ☐ ☐ _____
    Wet the mitt and apply soap. Wash the person's back
    and buttocks, moving from top to bottom and using
    long, firm strokes. Rinse thoroughly and pat the
    person's back and buttocks dry using a bath towel.
    At this point, a back massage may be given.

28. If the person is able to perform perineal care, assist   ☐ ☐ _____
    the person into Fowler's position and adjust the
    over-bed table so that the bathing supplies are within
    easy reach. Place the call-light control within easy
    reach and ask the person to signal when perineal care
    is complete. If the person is unable to perform
    perineal care, assist the person onto his back and
    complete perineal care.

29. Remove your gloves and dispose of them in a   ☐ ☐ _____
    facility-approved waste container. Put on a clean
    pair of gloves.

30. Help the person to apply lotion, powder, deodorant,   ☐ ☐ _____
    antiperspirant, or other personal care products as the
    person requests.

31. Help the person into the clean clothing.   ☐ ☐ _____

32. If the bedding is wet or soiled, change the bed linens.   ☐ ☐ _____

33. Carry out range-of-motion exercises as ordered.   ☐ ☐ _____

34. If the side rails are in use, return the side rails to the   ☐ ☐ _____
    raised position. Raise or lower the head of the bed as
    the person requests. Make sure that the bed is
    lowered to its lowest position and that the wheels are
    locked.

35. Gather the soiled linens and place them in the linen   ☐ ☐ _____
    hamper or linen bag. Dispose of disposable items in a
    facility-approved waste container. Clean equipment
    and return it to the storage area.

36. Remove your gloves and dispose of them in a   ☐ ☐ _____
    facility-approved waste container.

Finishing Up

37. Complete the "Finishing Up" steps.   ☐ ☐ _____

CHAPTER 19 PROCEDURE CHECKLISTS

PROCEDURE 19-1
Assisting the Nurse With a Dressing Change

Getting Ready	S	U	COMMENTS
1. Complete the "Getting Ready" steps.	☐	☐	_____

Procedure

	S	U	COMMENTS
2. Cover the over-bed table with paper towels or the bed protector. Place the dressing supplies on the over-bed table. Fold the top edges of the plastic bag down to make a cuff. Place the cuffed bag on the over-bed table.	☐	☐	_____
3. Make sure that the bed is positioned at a comfortable working height (to promote good body mechanics) and that the wheels are locked. If the side rails are in use, lower the side rail on the working side of the bed. The side rail on the opposite side of the bed should remain up.	☐	☐	_____
4. Help the person to a comfortable position that allows access to the wound.	☐	☐	_____
5. Fanfold the top linens to the foot of the bed. Adjust the person's hospital gown or pajamas as necessary to expose the wound.	☐	☐	_____
6. Put on the mask, gown, or both, if necessary. Put on the gloves.	☐	☐	_____
7. The nurse will remove the old dressing. The nurse may ask you to take the old dressing and place it in the cuffed plastic bag. Be careful to keep the soiled side of the dressing out of the person's sight. Do not let the dressing touch the outside of the plastic bag.	☐	☐	_____
8. Remove your gloves and dispose of them in a facility-approved waste container.	☐	☐	_____
9. Wait while the nurse inspects the wound and measures it, if necessary.	☐	☐	_____
10. Put on a clean pair of gloves.	☐	☐	_____
11. Assist as the nurse applies a new dressing.			
a. Open the wrapper containing the dressing and hold it open so that the nurse can remove the dressing. Do not touch the dressing. Dispose of the wrapper in a facility-approved waste container.	☐	☐	_____
b. If the dressing will be secured with tape, cut four pieces of tape for securing the dressing. For a 4 × 4 dressing, each piece of tape should measure 8 inches long. Hang the tape from the edge of the over-bed table.	☐	☐	_____

   c. If the nurse asks you to, use the tape strips to secure the dressing by placing one piece of tape along each side of the dressing. Center each piece of tape equally over the dressing and the person's skin.   ☐ ☐ _____

12. Remove your gloves (and gown and mask, if using) and dispose of them in a facility-approved waste container. Wash your hands.   ☐ ☐ _____

13. Re-cover the wound with the hospital gown or pajamas. Help the person back into a comfortable position, straighten the bottom linens, and draw the top linens over the person.   ☐ ☐ _____

14. Make sure that the bed is lowered to its lowest position and that the wheels are locked. If the side rails are in use, return the side rail to the raised position on the working side of the bed.   ☐ ☐ _____

15. Dispose of disposable items in a facility-approved waste container. Clean equipment and return it to the storage area.   ☐ ☐ _____

Finishing Up

16. Complete the "Finishing Up" steps.   ☐ ☐ _____

CHAPTER 20 PROCEDURE CHECKLISTS

PROCEDURE 20-1
Assisting With Hand Care

Getting Ready

	S	U	COMMENTS
1. Complete the "Getting Ready" steps.	☐	☐	_____

Procedure

	S	U	COMMENTS
2. Make sure that the bed is lowered to its lowest position and that the wheels are locked.	☐	☐	_____
3. Cover the over-bed table with paper towels. Pour some liquid soap into the emesis basin and fill the basin with warm water (100°F [37.7°C] to 115°F [46.1°C] on the bath thermometer). Place the emesis basin on the over-bed table, along with the nail care supplies and clean linens.	☐	☐	_____
4. If the side rails are in use, lower the side rail on the working side of the bed. The side rail on the opposite side of the bed should remain up.	☐	☐	_____
5. Help the person to transfer from the bed to a bedside chair, assist the person to sit on the edge of the bed, or raise the head of the bed as tolerated.	☐	☐	_____
6. Put on the gloves if contact with broken skin is likely.	☐	☐	_____
7. If the person is wearing nail polish and wants it removed, remove the nail polish by putting a small amount of nail polish remover on a cotton ball and gently rubbing each nail.	☐	☐	_____
8. Help the person to position the tips of her fingers in the basin to soak. Let the person soak her fingers for about 5 minutes.	☐	☐	_____
9. Working with one hand at a time, lift the person's hand out of the basin and wash the entire hand, including between the fingers, with the soapy washcloth. Use the orange stick to gently clean underneath the person's fingernails. Rinse thoroughly and pat the person's hand dry with a towel. Be sure to dry between the fingers. Repeat with the other hand.	☐	☐	_____
10. Remove the emesis basin and dry the person's hands thoroughly. If facility policy allows it, gently push the cuticles back with the orange stick.	☐	☐	_____
11. If facility policy allows it, use the nail clippers to cut the person's fingernails. If the person's nails need to be trimmed but this task is outside of your scope of practice, report this need to the nurse.	☐	☐	_____

12. Use the emery board to file the fingernails into an oval shape and smooth the rough edges. ☐ ☐ _____

13. Apply lotion to the person's hands and gently massage it into the skin. ☐ ☐ _____

14. Apply nail polish as the person requests. ☐ ☐ _____

15. If necessary, help the person return to bed. If the side rails are in use, return the side rails to the raised position. Lower the head of the bed as the person requests. ☐ ☐ _____

16. Gather the soiled linens and place them in the linen hamper or linen bag. Dispose of disposable items in a facility-approved waste container. Clean equipment and return it to the storage area. ☐ ☐ _____

17. Remove your gloves and dispose of them in a facility-approved waste container. ☐ ☐ _____

Finishing Up

18. Complete the "Finishing Up" steps. ☐ ☐ _____

PROCEDURE 20-2
Assisting With Foot Care

Getting Ready	S	U	COMMENTS
1. Complete the "Getting Ready" steps.	☐	☐	_____

Procedure

	S	U	COMMENTS
2. Make sure that the bed is lowered to its lowest position and that the wheels are locked.	☐	☐	_____
3. Cover the over-bed table with paper towels. Pour some liquid soap into the wash basin and fill the basin with warm water (100°F [37.7°C] to 115°F [46.1°C] on the bath thermometer). Place the wash basin on the over-bed table, along with the nail care supplies and clean linens.	☐	☐	_____
4. If the side rails are in use, lower the side rail on the working side of the bed. The side rail on the opposite side of the bed should remain up.	☐	☐	_____
5. If the person is able to get out of bed, help the person to transfer from the bed to a bedside chair. If the person is not able to get out of bed, raise the head of the bed as tolerated. Fanfold the top linens to the foot of the bed.	☐	☐	_____
6. Put on the gloves if contact with broken skin is likely.	☐	☐	_____
7. If the person is wearing nail polish and wants it removed, remove the nail polish by putting a small amount of nail polish remover on a cotton ball and gently rubbing each nail.	☐	☐	_____
8. Place a bed protector on the floor in front of the chair (if the person is out of bed) or on the bottom sheet (if the person is in bed). Place the wash basin on the bed protector.	☐	☐	_____
9. Help the person to position his feet in the basin to soak. Let the person soak his feet for about 5 minutes.	☐	☐	_____
10. Working with one foot at a time, lift the person's foot out of the basin and wash the entire foot, including between the toes, with the soapy washcloth. Apply soap to the nailbrush and gently scrub any rough areas. Use the orange stick to gently clean underneath the person's toenails. Rinse thoroughly and pat the person's foot dry with a towel. Be sure to dry between the toes. Repeat with the other foot.	☐	☐	_____
11. If facility policy allows it, use the nail clippers to cut the person's toenails. If the person's nails need to be trimmed but this task is outside of your scope of practice, report this need to the nurse.	☐	☐	_____

12. Use the emery board to smooth the rough edges of the toenails. ☐ ☐ _____

13. Apply lotion to the person's feet and gently massage it into the skin. ☐ ☐ _____

14. Apply nail polish as the person requests. ☐ ☐ _____

15. If necessary, help the person return to bed. If the side rails are in use, return the side rails to the raised position. Lower the head of the bed as the person requests. ☐ ☐ _____

16. Gather the soiled linens and place them in the linen hamper or linen bag. Dispose of disposable items in a facility-approved waste container. Clean equipment and return it to the storage area. ☐ ☐ _____

Finishing Up

17. Complete the "Finishing Up" steps. ☐ ☐ _____

PROCEDURE 20-3
Assisting a Person With Dressing

Getting Ready

	S	U	COMMENTS
1. Complete the "Getting Ready" steps.	☐	☐	_____

Procedure

	S	U	COMMENTS
2. Make sure that the bed is positioned at a comfortable working height (to promote good body mechanics) and that the wheels are locked.	☐	☐	_____
3. Lower the head of the bed so that the bed is flat (as tolerated). If the side rails are in use, lower the side rail on the working side of the bed. The side rail on the opposite side of the bed should remain up.	☐	☐	_____
4. Put on the gloves if contact with broken skin is likely.	☐	☐	_____
5. Spread the bath blanket over the top linens (and the person). If the person is able, have her hold the bath blanket. If not, tuck the corners under the person's shoulders. Fanfold the top linens to the foot of the bed.	☐	☐	_____

6. Assist the person with undressing:

	S	U	COMMENTS
a. **Garments that fasten in the back.** Undo any fasteners, such as buttons, zippers, snaps, or ties. Gently lift the person's head and shoulders and gather the garment around the person's neck. Working with the person's strongest side first, gently remove the arm from the garment by sliding the garment down the arm. Repeat with the other arm. (If it is not possible to lift the person's head and shoulders, roll the person onto his or her side facing away from you. Working with the person's strongest side first, gently remove the arm from the garment. Roll the person onto her other side, facing you and remove the other arm from the garment.) Remove the garment completely by lifting it over the person's head.	☐	☐	_____
b. **Garments that fasten in the front.** Undo any fasteners, such as buttons, zippers, snaps, or ties. To remove the top, gently lift the person's head and shoulders. Working with the person's strongest side first, gently remove the arm from the garment by sliding the garment over the shoulder and down the arm. Gather the garment behind the person and remove the garment completely by sliding the other sleeve over the weak shoulder and arm. To remove the bottoms, undo any fasteners, such as buttons, zippers or snaps. Ask the person to lift her buttocks off the bed and gently slide the pants down to the ankles	☐	☐	_____

and over the feet. (If the person cannot raise her buttocks off the bed, help the person to roll first to her strong side, allowing you to pull the bottoms down on the weak side. Then roll the person to her weak side and finish pulling the bottoms down.)

□ □ _____

7. Assist the person with putting on her undergarments:

a. **Underpants.** Facing the foot of the bed, gather the underpants together at the leg opening and at the waistband. Working with one foot at a time, slip first one foot and then the other through the waistband and into the leg openings. Slide the underpants up the person's legs as far as they will go, and then ask the person to lift her buttocks off the bed. Gently slide the underpants up over the buttocks. (If the person cannot raise her buttocks off the bed, help the person to roll first to her strong side, allowing you to pull the underpants up on the weak side. Then roll the person to her weak side and finish pulling the underpants up.) Adjust the underpants so that they fit comfortably.

□ □ _____

b. **Bra.** Working with the person's weak side first, slip the arms through the straps and position the straps on the shoulders so that the front of the bra is covering the person's chest. Adjust the cups of the bra over the person's breasts. Raise the person's head and shoulders and help the person to lean forward so that you can fasten the bra in the back.

□ □ _____

c. **Undershirt.** Facing the head of the bed, gather the top and the bottom of the undershirt together at the neck opening. Place the undershirt over the person's head. Working with the person's weak side first, slip the arms through the arm openings. Raise the person's head and shoulders and help the person to lean forward so that you can pull the undershirt down, smoothing out any wrinkles.

□ □ _____

8. Assist the person with putting on her outerwear:

a. **Pants.** Assist the person with putting on her pants by following the same procedure as that used for putting on underpants (see step 7a). Fasten any buttons, zippers, snaps, or ties.

□ □ _____

b. **Shirts and sweaters that fasten in the front.** Facing the head of the bed, place your hand and arm through the wristband of the garment. Working with the person's weak side first, grasp the person's hand and slip the garment off of your hand and arm, gently guiding the person's arm into the sleeve. Pull the sleeve up, adjusting it at the shoulder. Raise the person's head and shoulders and help the person to lean forward so

□ □ _____

that you can bring the other side of the garment around the back of the person's body. Guide the person's strong arm into the sleeve of the garment. Fasten any buttons, zippers, snaps, or ties.

   c. **Sweatshirts and pullover sweaters.** Assist the person with putting on a sweatshirt or pullover sweater by following the same procedure as that used for putting on an undershirt (see step 7c). Fasten any buttons, zippers, snaps, or ties. ☐ ☐ _____

   d. **Blouses that fasten in the back.** Facing the head of the bed, place your hand and arm through the wristband of the garment. Working with the person's weak side first, grasp the person's hand and slip the garment off of your hand and arm, gently guiding the person's arm into the sleeve. Pull the sleeve up, adjusting it at the shoulder. Repeat for the other side. Raise the person's head and shoulders and help the person to lean forward so that you can bring the sides of the garment around to the back. Fasten any buttons, zippers, snaps, or ties. ☐ ☐ _____

9. Assist the person with putting on footwear:

   a. **Socks or knee-high stockings.** Gather the sock or stocking, bringing the toe area and the opening together. With the toe area facing up, slip the sock or stocking over the person's foot. Smooth the heel of the sock or stocking over the person's heel, and pull the sock or stocking up into position. Adjust the sock or stocking so that it fits comfortably. Repeat for the other foot. ☐ ☐ _____

   b. **Shoes or slippers.** If the shoe has laces, loosen them completely to make it easier to slip the shoe onto the foot. Guide the person's foot into the shoe or slipper. A shoehorn may be used to help ease the person's heel into the shoe. Make sure that the foot is seated properly in the shoe. Socks or stockings should not be bunched at the toe. If necessary, tie the shoe or fasten the Velcro™ fasteners securely. ☐ ☐ _____

10. If the person will be remaining in bed and the side rails are in use, return the side rails to the raised position. Raise the head of the bed as the person requests. ☐ ☐ _____

11. Gather the soiled garments and place them in the linen hamper or linen bag. ☐ ☐ _____

12. Remove your gloves and dispose of them in a facility-approved waste container. ☐ ☐ _____

Finishing Up

13. Complete the "Finishing Up" steps. ☐ ☐ _____

PROCEDURE 20-4
Changing a Hospital Gown

Getting Ready	S	U	COMMENTS
1. Complete the "Getting Ready" steps.	☐	☐	_____

Procedure

	S	U	COMMENTS
2. Make sure that the bed is positioned at a comfortable working height (to promote good body mechanics) and that the wheels are locked.	☐	☐	_____
3. Lower the head of the bed so that the bed is flat (as tolerated). If the side rails are in use, lower them on the working side of the bed. The side rails on the opposite side of the bed should remain up.	☐	☐	_____
4. Put on the gloves if contact with broken skin is likely.	☐	☐	_____
5. Have the person turn onto her side facing away from you so that you can untie the gown at the neck and waist. Assist the person back into the supine position. If the person cannot turn onto her side, reach under the person and untie the gown.	☐	☐	_____
6. Loosen the gown from around the person's body.	☐	☐	_____
7. Unfold the clean gown and lay it over the person's chest.	☐	☐	_____
8. Working with the person's strongest side first, remove one sleeve at a time, leaving the old gown draped over the person's body.	☐	☐	_____
9. Working with the person's weakest side first, slide the arm through the sleeve of the clean gown. Repeat for the other arm.	☐	☐	_____
10. Remove the soiled gown from underneath the clean gown and place it in the linen hamper or linen bag.	☐	☐	_____
11. Have the person turn onto her side, facing away from you, so that you can tie the gown at the neck and waist (or reach under the person and tie the gown). Adjust the gown so that it fits comfortably.	☐	☐	_____
12. If the side rails are in use, return the side rails to the raised position. Raise the head of the bed as the person requests.	☐	☐	_____
13. Remove your gloves and dispose of them in a facility-approved waste container.	☐	☐	_____

Finishing Up

	S	U	COMMENTS
14. Complete the "Finishing Up" steps.	☐	☐	_____

PROCEDURE 20-5
Shampooing a Person's Hair in Bed

Getting Ready	S	U	COMMENTS
1. Complete the "Getting Ready" steps.	☐	☐	_____

Procedure

	S	U	COMMENTS
2. Make sure that the bed is positioned at a comfortable working height (to promote good body mechanics) and that the wheels are locked.	☐	☐	_____
3. Fill the water pitcher with warm water (100°F [37.7°C] to 115°F [46.1°C] on the bath thermometer).	☐	☐	_____
4. Cover the over-bed table with paper towels. Place the hair care supplies and clean linens on the over-bed table.	☐	☐	_____
5. Raise the head of the bed as tolerated. Comb the person's hair to remove snarls and tangles.	☐	☐	_____
6. Lower the head of the bed so that the bed is flat (as tolerated). If the side rails are in use, lower the side rail on the working side of the bed. The side rail on the opposite side of the bed should remain up.	☐	☐	_____
7. Put on the gloves if contact with broken skin is likely.	☐	☐	_____
8. Gently lift the person's head and shoulders and reposition the pillow under the person's shoulders. Cover the head of the bed and the pillow with the bed protector and place the shampoo trough on the bed protector. Help the person to rest her head on the shampoo trough. Place a towel across the person's shoulders and chest.	☐	☐	_____
9. Place the wash basin on the floor beside the bed to catch the water as it drains from the shampoo trough.	☐	☐	_____
10. Ask the person to hold the washcloth over her eyes.	☐	☐	_____
11. Holding the water pitcher in one hand, slowly pour water over the person's hair until the hair is completely wet. Use your other hand to help direct the flow of water away from the person's eyes and ears.	☐	☐	_____
12. Apply a small amount of shampoo to the wet hair. Lather the hair and massage the scalp to help stimulate the circulation.	☐	☐	_____
13. Using the water pitcher, rinse the hair thoroughly.	☐	☐	_____
14. Apply conditioner, as the person requests. Rinse the hair thoroughly.	☐	☐	_____
15. Gently lift the person's head and shoulders and remove the shampoo trough and bed protector. Wrap the person's hair in a towel.	☐	☐	_____

16. Raise the head of the bed as tolerated. Gently pat the person's face, neck, and ears dry and finish towel drying the hair.

☐ ☐ _____

17. Replace any wet or soiled linens. (If the side rails are in use, raise the side rails before leaving the bedside to get the necessary replacement linens.)

☐ ☐ _____

18. Comb the person's hair to remove snarls and tangles.

☐ ☐ _____

19. Dry and style the hair with the brush and blow dryer, as the person requests. Use the cool setting and take care not to burn the person's scalp or face.

☐ ☐ _____

20. Reposition the pillow under the person's head and straighten the bed linens. If the side rails are in use, return the side rails to the raised position. Lower the head of the bed as the person requests.

☐ ☐ _____

21. Gather the soiled linens and place them in the linen hamper or linen bag. Dispose of disposable items in a facility-approved waste container. Clean equipment and return it to the storage area.

☐ ☐ _____

22. Remove your gloves and dispose of them in a facility-approved waste container.

☐ ☐ _____

Finishing Up

23. Complete the "Finishing Up" steps.

☐ ☐ _____

PROCEDURE 20-6
Combing a Person's Hair

Getting Ready	S	U	COMMENTS
1. Complete the "Getting Ready" steps.	☐	☐	_____

Procedure

	S	U	COMMENTS
2. Make sure that the bed is positioned at a comfortable working height (to promote good body mechanics) and that the wheels are locked.	☐	☐	_____
3. Cover the over-bed table with paper towels. Place the hair care supplies and clean linens on the over-bed table.	☐	☐	_____
4. Raise the head of the bed as tolerated. Gently lift the person's head and shoulders and cover the pillow with a towel. Drape another towel across the person's back and shoulders.	☐	☐	_____
5. If the side rails are in use, lower the side rail on the working side of the bed. The side rail on the opposite side of the bed should remain up.	☐	☐	_____
6. If the hair is tangled, work on the tangles first. Put a small amount of detangler or leave-in conditioner on the tangled hair. Begin at the ends of the hair and work toward the scalp. Hold the lock of hair just above the tangle (closest to the scalp) and use the wide-tooth comb to gently work through the tangle.	☐	☐	_____
7. Using the brush and working with one 2-inch section at a time, gently brush the hair, moving from the roots of the hair toward the ends.	☐	☐	_____
8. Secure the hair using barrettes, clips, or pins or braid the hair, as the person requests. Offer the person the mirror to check her appearance when you are finished. Remove the towels from the pillow and the person's shoulders.	☐	☐	_____
9. Reposition the pillow under the person's head and straighten the bed linens. If the side rails are in use, return the side rails to the raised position. Lower the head of the bed as the person requests.	☐	☐	_____
10. Gather the soiled linens and place them in the linen hamper or linen bag. Dispose of disposable items in a facility-approved waste container. Clean equipment and return it to the storage area.	☐	☐	_____

Finishing Up

	S	U	COMMENTS
11. Complete the "Finishing Up" steps.	☐	☐	_____

PROCEDURE 20-7
Shaving a Person's Face

	S	U	COMMENTS

Getting Ready

1. Complete the "Getting Ready" steps.   ☐ ☐ _____

Procedure

2. Make sure that the bed is lowered to its lowest position and that the wheels are locked. ☐ ☐ _____

3. Fill the wash basin with warm water (100°F [37.7°C] to 115°F [46.1°C] on the bath thermometer). ☐ ☐ _____

4. Cover the over-bed table with paper towels. Place the wash basin, shaving supplies, and clean linens on the over-bed table. ☐ ☐ _____

5. If the side rails are in use, lower the side rail on the working side of the bed. The side rail on the opposite side of the bed should remain up. ☐ ☐ _____

6. Help the person to transfer from the bed to a bedside chair, assist the person to sit on the edge of the bed, or raise the head of the bed as tolerated. ☐ ☐ _____

7. Place a towel across the person's shoulders and chest. ☐ ☐ _____

8. Put on the gloves. ☐ ☐ _____

9. Wet the washcloth with warm, clean water. Soften the beard by holding the washcloth against the person's face for 2 to 3 minutes. ☐ ☐ _____

10. Apply shaving cream, gel, or soap to the beard. ☐ ☐ _____

11. Shave the person's cheeks:

   a. Stand facing the person. ☐ ☐ _____

   b. Gently pull the skin tight and shave downward, in the direction of hair growth (i.e., toward the chin). Use short, even strokes, rinsing the razor frequently in the wash basin. Repeat until all of the lather on the cheek has been removed. ☐ ☐ _____

   c. Repeat for the other cheek. ☐ ☐ _____

12. Shave the person's chin:

   a. Ask the person to "tighten the chin" by drawing the lower lip over the teeth. ☐ ☐ _____

   b. Shave the chin using short, even, downward strokes. Repeat until all of the lather on the chin has been removed, rinsing the razor frequently in the wash basin. ☐ ☐ _____

13. Shave the person's neck:

   a. Ask the person to tip his head back. ☐ ☐ _____

   b. Gently pull the skin tight and shave upward, in the direction of hair growth (i.e., toward the chin). Use short, even strokes, rinsing the razor frequently in the wash basin. Repeat until all of the lather on the neck has been removed.

14. Shave the area between the person's nose and upper lip:
    a. Ask the person to "tighten his upper lip" by drawing the upper lip over the teeth. ☐ ☐ _____
    b. Shave the area between the nose and the upper lip using short, even downward strokes. Repeat until all of the lather has been removed, rinsing the razor frequently in the wash basin. ☐ ☐ _____

15. Change the water in the wash basin. (If the side rails are in use, raise the side rails before leaving the bedside.) Form a mitt around your hand with the washcloth and wet the mitt with warm, clean water. Wash the person's face and neck. Rinse thoroughly and pat the person's face, neck, and ears dry with the face towel. ☐ ☐ _____

16. Apply aftershave lotion, as the person requests. ☐ ☐ _____

17. If you have accidentally nicked the skin and the person is bleeding, apply direct pressure with a tissue until the bleeding stops. Report the incident to the nurse. ☐ ☐ _____

18. If necessary, help the person return to bed. If the side rails are in use, return the side rails to the raised position. ☐ ☐ _____

19. Gather the soiled linens and place them in the linen hamper or linen bag. Dispose of disposable items in a facility-approved waste container. Clean equipment and return it to the storage area. ☐ ☐ _____

20. Remove your gloves and dispose of them in a facility-approved waste container. ☐ ☐ _____

Finishing Up

21. Complete the "Finishing Up" steps. ☐ ☐ _____

CHAPTER 21 PROCEDURE CHECKLISTS

PROCEDURE 21-1
Feeding a Dependent Person

Getting Ready

	S	U	COMMENTS
1. Complete the "Getting Ready" steps.	☐	☐	_____

Procedure

	S	U	COMMENTS
2. Cover the over-bed table with paper towels. Place the oral hygiene supplies on the over-bed table. Fill the wash basin with warm water (110°F [37.7°C] to 115°F [46.1°C] on the bath thermometer). Place the basin on the over-bed table.	☐	☐	_____
3. If the side rails are in use, lower the side rail on the working side of the bed. The side rail on the opposite side of the bed should remain up. Raise the head of the bed. Make sure that the bed is positioned at a comfortable working height (to promote good body mechanics) and that the wheels are locked.	☐	☐	_____
4. Put on the gloves.	☐	☐	_____
5. Assist the person with oral hygiene.	☐	☐	_____
6. Offer the bedpan or urinal. If the person uses the bedpan or urinal, empty and clean it before proceeding with the meal. Remove your gloves and dispose of them in a facility-approved waste container. Wash your hands.	☐	☐	_____
7. Wash the person's hands and face.	☐	☐	_____
8. Clear the over-bed table and position it over the bed at the proper height for the person.	☐	☐	_____
9. Get the meal tray from the dietary cart. (If the side rails are in use, raise the side rails before leaving the bedside.) Check the meal tray to make sure that it has the person's name on it and that it contains the correct diet for the person. Place the meal tray on the over-bed table.			
10. Ask the person if he would like to use a clothing protector. Put the clothing protector on the person, if desired.	☐	☐	_____
11. Uncover the meal tray and prepare the food for eating (for example, cut the meat, butter the bread, open any containers). Tell the person what is on the tray.	☐	☐	_____
12. Take a seat.	☐	☐	_____
13. Allow the person to choose what he would like to taste first. Using a spoon, offer a small bite to the person (fill the spoon no more than one-third full). Allow the person enough time to swallow the food.	☐	☐	_____

14. Offer the person something to drink every few bites. Use the napkin to wipe the person's mouth and chin as often as necessary. Allow the person to assist with the eating process to the best of his ability. ☐ ☐ _____

15. Continue in this manner until the person is finished. Encourage the person to finish the food on the tray, but do not force the person to eat. ☐ ☐ _____

16. Remove the tray and the clothing protector when the person has finished eating. ☐ ☐ _____

17. Put on a clean pair of gloves. Assist the person with oral hygiene. ☐ ☐ _____

18. If the side rails are in use, return the side rails to the raised position. Lower the head of the bed as the person requests. Make sure that the bed is lowered to its lowest position and that the wheels are locked. ☐ ☐ _____

19. Gather the soiled linens and place them in the linen hamper or linen bag. Dispose of disposable items in a facility-approved waste container. Clean equipment and return it to the storage area. ☐ ☐ _____

20. Remove your gloves and dispose of them in a facility-approved waste container. ☐ ☐ _____

21. Record the percentage of food eaten and the amount of fluid intake in the person's medical record, per your facility's policy. Report an abnormal appetite to the nurse (for example, less than 70 percent of the total meal consumed). ☐ ☐ _____

Finishing Up

22. Complete the "Finishing Up" steps. ☐ ☐ _____

CHAPTER 22 PROCEDURE CHECKLISTS

PROCEDURE 22-1
Assisting a Person With Using a Bedpan

Getting Ready

	S	U	COMMENTS
1. Complete the "Getting Ready" steps.	☐	☐	_____

Procedure

	S	U	COMMENTS
2. Make sure that the bed is positioned at a comfortable working height (to promote good body mechanics) and that the wheels are locked. If the side rails are in use, lower the side rail on the working side of the bed. The side rail on the opposite side of the bed should remain up. If necessary, lower the head of the bed so that the bed is flat (as tolerated).	☐	☐	_____
3. Put on the gloves.	☐	☐	_____
4. Fanfold the top linens to the foot of the bed. Place the bed protector on the bed. Adjust the person's hospital gown or pajama bottoms as necessary to expose the person's buttocks.	☐	☐	_____
5. Place the bedpan underneath the person's buttocks. This can be accomplished by either helping the person to lie on her side, facing away from you, or by asking the person to bend her knees, lift her buttocks, and press her heels into the mattress. Slide the bedpan underneath the person (if the person is holding her buttocks away from the bed by bending her knees) or place the bedpan against her buttocks and help her to roll back onto it.			
a. A standard bedpan is positioned like a regular toilet seat.	☐	☐	_____
b. A fracture pan is positioned with the narrow end pointed toward the head of the bed.	☐	☐	_____
6. Raise the head of the bed as tolerated. Draw the top linens over the person for modesty and warmth.	☐	☐	_____
7. Make sure that the toilet paper and the call-light control are within reach. If the side rails are in use, return the side rails to the raised position.	☐	☐	_____
8. Remove your gloves and wash your hands.	☐	☐	_____
9. If safety permits, leave the room and ask the person to call you when she is finished. Remember to close the door on your way out.	☐	☐	_____
10. Return when the person signals. Remember to knock before entering.	☐	☐	_____
11. If the side rails are in use, lower the side rail on the working side of the bed. Lower the head of the bed so that the bed is flat (as tolerated).	☐	☐	_____

12. Put on a clean pair of gloves.   ☐ ☐ _____

13. Fanfold the top linens to the foot of the bed.   ☐ ☐ _____

14. Ask the person to bend her knees, lift her buttocks, and press her heels into the mattress so that you can remove the bedpan and bed protector. (Or help the person to roll onto her side, facing away from you, while you hold the bedpan securely in place against the mattress to prevent the contents from spilling. Remove the bedpan and bed protector and then help the person to roll back.) If necessary, help the person to use the toilet paper.   ☐ ☐ _____

15. Cover the bedpan with the bedpan cover or paper towels. Take the bedpan to the bathroom. (If the side rails are in use, raise them before leaving the bedside.)   ☐ ☐ _____

16. Remove your gloves and dispose of them in a facility-approved waste container. Wash your hands.   ☐ ☐ _____

17. Return to the bedside. Give the person a wet washcloth and help the person to wash her hands. Make sure the person's perineum is clean and dry. If necessary, provide perineal care.   ☐ ☐ _____

18. Adjust the person's hospital gown or pajama bottoms as necessary to cover the buttocks. Help the person back into a comfortable position, straighten the bottom linens, and draw the top linens over the person. Raise the head of the bed, as the person requests. Make sure that the bed is lowered to its lowest position and that the wheels are locked.   ☐ ☐ _____

19. Return to the bathroom. Put on a clean pair of gloves. If the person is on intake and output (I&O) status, measure the urine. Note the color, amount, and quality of the urine or feces before emptying the contents of the bedpan into the toilet. (If anything unusual is observed, do not empty the bedpan until a nurse has had a chance to look at its contents.)   ☐ ☐ _____

20. Gather the soiled linens and place them in the linen hamper or linen bag. Dispose of disposable items in a facility-approved waste container. Clean equipment and return it to the storage area.   ☐ ☐ _____

21. Remove your gloves and dispose of them in a facility-approved waste container.   ☐ ☐ _____

Finishing Up

22. Complete the "Finishing Up" steps.   ☐ ☐ _____

PROCEDURE 22-2
Assisting a Man With Using a Urinal

	S	U	COMMENTS

Getting Ready

1. Complete the "Getting Ready" steps. □ □ _____

Procedure

2. Ask the man what position he prefers—lying, sitting, or standing. If necessary, raise the head of the bed as tolerated. If the man would prefer to stand, help him to sit on the edge of the bed and then to stand up. □ □ _____

3. Put on the gloves. □ □ _____

4. Hand the man the urinal. If necessary, assist him in positioning it correctly. □ □ _____

5. Make sure that the toilet paper and the call-light control are within reach. □ □ _____

6. Remove your gloves and wash your hands. □ □ _____

7. If safety permits, leave the room and ask the man to call you when he is finished. Remember to close the door on your way out. □ □ _____

8. Return when the man signals. Remember to knock before entering. □ □ _____

9. Put on a clean pair of gloves. Have the man hand you the urinal, or remove it if he is unable to hand it to you. Put the lid on the urinal and hang it on the side rail while you assist the man with handwashing and perineal care as needed. Lower the head of the bed as the man requests. □ □ _____

10. Take the urinal to the bathroom. If the man is on intake and output (I&O) status, measure the urine. Note the color, amount, and quality of the urine before emptying the contents of the urinal into the toilet. (If anything unusual is observed, do not empty the urinal until a nurse has had a chance to look at its contents.) □ □ _____

11. Gather the soiled linens and place them in the linen hamper or linen bag. Dispose of disposable items in a facility-approved waste container. Clean equipment and return it to the storage area. □ □ _____

12. Remove your gloves and dispose of them in a facility-approved waste container. □ □ _____

Finishing Up

13. Complete the "Finishing Up" steps. □ □ _____

PROCEDURE 22-3
Providing Catheter Care

Getting Ready	S	U	COMMENTS
1. Complete the "Getting Ready" steps.	☐	☐	_____

Procedure

	S	U	COMMENTS
2. Cover the over-bed table with paper towels.	☐	☐	_____
3. Lower the head of the bed so that the bed is flat (as tolerated). Make sure that the bed is positioned at a comfortable working height (to promote good body mechanics) and that the wheels are locked.	☐	☐	_____
4. Fill the wash basin with warm water (110°F [43.3°C] to 115°F [46.1°C] on the bath thermometer). Place the wash basin, soap, towels, and washcloths on the over-bed table.	☐	☐	_____
5. If the side rails are in use, lower the side rail on the working side of the bed. The side rail on the opposite side of the bed should remain up.	☐	☐	_____
6. Put on the gloves.	☐	☐	_____
7. Spread the bath blanket over the top linens (and the person). If the person is able, have him hold the bath blanket. If not, tuck the corners under the person's shoulders. Fanfold the top linens to the foot of the bed.	☐	☐	_____
8. Adjust the person's hospital gown or pajama bottoms as necessary to expose the person's perineum.	☐	☐	_____
9. Ask the person to open his legs and bend his knees, if possible. If the person is not able to bend his knees, help the person to spread his legs as much as possible.	☐	☐	_____
10. Position the bath blanket over the person so that one corner can be wrapped under and around each leg.	☐	☐	_____
11. Position a bed protector under the person's buttocks to keep the bed linens dry.	☐	☐	_____
12. Lift the corner of the bath blanket that is between the person's legs upward, exposing only the perineal area.	☐	☐	_____
13. Form a mitt around your hand with one of the washcloths. Wet the mitt with warm, clean water and apply soap or antiseptic solution.			
a. **If the person is a woman:** Using the other hand, separate the labia. Place your washcloth-covered hand at the top of the vulva and stroke downward to the anus. Repeat, using a different part of the washcloth each time, until the area is clean. Rinse and dry the vulva and perineum thoroughly.	☐	☐	_____

   b. If the person is a circumcised man: Place your washcloth-covered hand at the tip of the penis and wash in a circular motion, downward to the base of the penis. Repeat, using a different part of the washcloth each time, until the area is clean. Rinse and dry the tip and the shaft of the penis thoroughly.   ☐ ☐ _____

   c. If the person is an uncircumcised man: Retract the foreskin by gently pushing the skin toward the base of the penis. Place your washcloth-covered hand at the tip of the penis and wash in a circular motion, downward to the base of the penis. Repeat, using a different part of the washcloth each time, until the area is clean. Rinse and dry the tip and the shaft of the penis thoroughly before gently pulling the foreskin back into its normal position.   ☐ ☐ _____

14. Using a clean part of the washcloth, clean the catheter tubing, starting at the body and moving outward from the body about four inches. Hold the catheter near the opening of the urethra. This will help to prevent tugging on the catheter as you clean it.   ☐ ☐ _____

15. Dry the perineal area thoroughly using a towel.   ☐ ☐ _____

16. Check that the catheter tubing is free from kinks. Make sure that it is securely taped to the person's leg.   ☐ ☐ _____

17. Remove your gloves and dispose of them in a facility-approved waste container.   ☐ ☐ _____

18. Assist the person into the supine position. Remove the bath blanket, and help the person into the clean clothing.   ☐ ☐ _____

19. If the side rails are in use, return the side rails to the raised position. Raise the head of the bed as the person requests. Make sure that the bed is lowered to its lowest position and that the wheels are locked.   ☐ ☐ _____

20. Gather the soiled linens and place them in the linen hamper or linen bag. Dispose of disposable items in a facility-approved waste container. Clean equipment and return it to the storage area.   ☐ ☐ _____

Finishing Up

21. Complete the "Finishing Up" steps.   ☐ ☐ _____

PROCEDURE 22-4
Emptying a Urine Drainage Bag

Getting Ready	S	U	COMMENTS
1. Complete the "Getting Ready" steps.	☐	☐	_____

Procedure

	S	U	COMMENTS
2. Put on the gloves.	☐	☐	_____
3. Place a paper towel on the floor, underneath the urine drainage bag. Unhook the drainage bag emptying spout from its holder on the urine drainage bag. Position the graduate on the paper towel underneath the emptying spout.	☐	☐	_____
4. Unclamp the emptying spout on the urine drainage bag and allow all of the urine to drain into the graduate. Avoid touching the tip of the emptying spout with your hands or the side of the graduate.	☐	☐	_____
5. After the urine has drained into the graduate, wipe the emptying spout with an alcohol wipe (or follow facility policy). Reclamp the emptying spout and return it to its holder.	☐	☐	_____
6. If the person is on intake and output (I&O) status, measure the urine. Note the color, amount, and quality of the urine before emptying the contents of the graduate into the toilet. (If anything unusual is observed, do not empty the graduate until a nurse has had a chance to look at its contents.)	☐	☐	_____
7. Dispose of disposable items in a facility-approved waste container. Clean equipment and return it to the storage area.	☐	☐	_____
8. Remove your gloves and dispose of them in a facility-approved waste container.	☐	☐	_____

Finishing Up

	S	U	COMMENTS
9. Complete the "Finishing Up" steps.	☐	☐	_____

PROCEDURE 22-5
Collecting a Routine Urine Specimen

Getting Ready	S	U	COMMENTS
1. Complete the "Getting Ready" steps.	☐	☐	_____

Procedure

	S	U	COMMENTS
2. Complete the label with the person's name, room number, and other identifying information. Put the completed label on the specimen container. Take the specimen container to the bathroom. Place a paper towel on the counter. Open the specimen container and place the lid on the paper towel, with the inside of the lid facing up.	☐	☐	_____
3. If the person will be using a regular toilet or bedside commode, fit the specimen collection device underneath the toilet or commode seat. Otherwise, provide the person with a bedpan or urinal, as applicable.	☐	☐	_____
4. Assist the person with urination as necessary. Before leaving the room, remind the person not to have a bowel movement or place toilet paper into the specimen collection device, bedpan, or urinal. Provide a plastic bag or waste container for the used toilet paper.	☐	☐	_____
5. Return when the person signals. Remember to knock before entering.	☐	☐	_____
6. Put on the gloves.	☐	☐	_____
7. If the person used a regular toilet or bedside commode, assist the person with handwashing and perineal care as necessary and then help the person to return to bed. If the person used a bedpan or urinal, cover and remove the bedpan or urinal and assist the person with handwashing and perineal care as necessary.	☐	☐	_____
8. Take the covered bedpan, urinal, or specimen collection device (if the person used a bedside commode) to the bathroom. (If the side rails are in use, raise the side rails before leaving the bedside.)	☐	☐	_____
9. If the person is on intake and output (I&O) status, measure the urine. Note the color, amount, and quality of the urine.	☐	☐	_____
10. Raise the toilet seat. While holding the specimen container over the toilet, carefully fill it about three-quarters full with urine from the specimen collection device, bedpan, or urinal. Discard the rest of the urine into the toilet.	☐	☐	_____
11. Put the lid on the specimen container. Make sure that the lid is tight. Put the specimen container on the paper towel on the counter.	☐	☐	_____

12. Remove one glove and dispose of it in a facility-approved waste container. Holding the plastic transport bag in your ungloved hand, place the specimen container into the transport bag with your gloved hand. Avoid touching the outside of the transport bag with your glove. ☐ ☐ _____

13. Remove the other glove and dispose of it in a facility-approved waste container. ☐ ☐ _____

14. Gather the soiled linens and place them in the linen hamper or linen bag. Dispose of disposable items in a facility-approved waste container. Clean equipment and return it to the storage area. ☐ ☐ _____

15. Take the specimen container to the designated location. ☐ ☐ _____

Finishing Up

16. Complete the "Finishing Up" steps. ☐ ☐ _____

PROCEDURE 22-6

Collecting a Midstream ("Clean Catch") Urine Specimen

	S	U	COMMENTS

Getting Ready

1. Complete the "Getting Ready" steps. ☐ ☐ _____

Procedure

2. Complete the label with the person's name, room number, and other identifying information. Put the completed label on the specimen container. ☐ ☐ _____

3. If the person will be using a regular toilet or bedside commode, help the person to the bathroom or bedside commode. Otherwise, provide the person with a bedpan or urinal, as applicable. ☐ ☐ _____

4. Put on the gloves. ☐ ☐ _____

5. Place a paper towel on the counter (if the person is in the bathroom) or on the over-bed table (if the person is using a bedside commode, bedpan, or urinal). Open the specimen container and place the lid on the paper towel, with the inside of the lid facing up. ☐ ☐ _____

6. Open the "clean catch" kit. Have the person clean his or her perineum using the wipes in the kit. Assist as necessary:

   a. **If the person is a woman:** Use one hand to separate the labia. Hold the wipe in the other hand. Place your wipe-covered hand at the top of the vulva and stroke downward to the anus. ☐ ☐ _____

   b. **If the person is a circumcised man:** Use one hand to hold the penis slightly away from the body. Hold the wipe in the other hand. Place your wipe-covered hand at the tip of the penis and wash in a circular motion, downward to the base of the penis. ☐ ☐ _____

   c. **If the person is an uncircumcised man:** Retract the foreskin by gently pushing the skin toward the base of the penis. Place your wipe-covered hand at the tip of the penis and wash in a circular motion, downward to the base of the penis. ☐ ☐ _____

7. Assist the person with urination as necessary. Before leaving the room:

   a. Make sure that the toilet paper, call-light control, and specimen cup are within reach. ☐ ☐ _____

   b. Remind the person that he or she must start the stream of urine, then stop it, then restart it. The urine sample is to be collected from the restarted flow. If the person is a woman, she must hold the labia open until the specimen is collected. If the person is an uncircumcised man, he must keep the foreskin pulled back until the specimen is collected. ☐ ☐ _____

8. Remove your gloves and dispose of them in a facility-approved waste container. ☐ ☐ _____

9. Return when the person signals. Remember to knock before entering. ☐ ☐ _____

10. Put on a clean pair of gloves. ☐ ☐ _____

11. If the person used a regular toilet or bedside commode, assist the person with handwashing and perineal care as necessary and then help the person to return to bed. If the person used a bedpan or urinal, remove the bedpan or urinal and assist the person with handwashing and perineal care as necessary. ☐ ☐ _____

12. Put the lid on the specimen container, being careful not to touch the inside of the lid or container. Make sure that the lid is tight. Put the specimen container on the paper towel on the counter or over-bed table. ☐ ☐ _____

13. Remove one glove and dispose of it in a facility-approved waste container. Holding the plastic transport bag in your ungloved hand, place the specimen container into the transport bag with your gloved hand. Avoid touching the outside of the transport bag with your glove. ☐ ☐ _____

14. Remove the other glove and dispose of it in a facility-approved waste container. ☐ ☐ _____

15. Gather the soiled linens and place them in the linen hamper or linen bag. Dispose of disposable items in a facility-approved waste container. Clean equipment and return it to the storage area. ☐ ☐ _____

16. Take the specimen container to the designated location. ☐ ☐ _____

Finishing Up

17. Complete the "Finishing Up" steps. ☐ ☐ _____

CHAPTER 23 PROCEDURE CHECKLISTS

PROCEDURE 23-1
Collecting a Stool Specimen

Getting Ready	S	U	COMMENTS
1. Complete the "Getting Ready" steps.	☐	☐	_____

Procedure

	S	U	COMMENTS
2. Complete the label with the person's name, room number, and other identifying information. Put the completed label on the specimen container. Take the specimen container to the bathroom. Place a paper towel on the counter. Open the specimen container and place the lid on the paper towel with the inside of the lid facing up.	☐	☐	_____
3. If the person will be using a regular toilet or bedside commode, fit the specimen collection device underneath the toilet or commode seat. Otherwise, provide the person with a bedpan.	☐	☐	_____
4. Assist the person with defecation as necessary. Before leaving the room, remind the person not to urinate or place toilet paper into the specimen collection device or bedpan. Provide a plastic bag or waste container for the used toilet paper.	☐	☐	_____
5. Return when the person signals. Remember to knock before entering.	☐	☐	_____
6. Put on the gloves.	☐	☐	_____
7. If the person used a regular toilet or bedside commode, assist the person with handwashing and then help the person to return to bed. Provide perineal care as necessary. If the person used a bedpan, cover and remove the bedpan and assist the person with handwashing and perineal care as necessary.	☐	☐	_____
8. Take the covered bedpan or specimen collection device (if the person used a bedside commode) to the bathroom. (If the side rails are in use, raise the side rails before leaving the bedside.)	☐	☐	_____
9. Note the color, amount, and quality of the feces. Using the tongue depressor, take two tablespoons of feces from the bedpan or specimen collection device and put them into the specimen container. Dispose of the tongue depressor in a facility-approved waste container. Empty the remaining contents of the bedpan or specimen collection device into the toilet.	☐	☐	_____
10. Put the lid on the specimen container. Make sure that the lid is tight. Put the specimen container on the paper towel on the counter.	☐	☐	_____

11. Remove one glove and dispose of it in a facility-approved waste container. Holding the plastic transport bag in your ungloved hand, place the specimen container into the transport bag with your gloved hand. Avoid touching the outside of the transport bag with your glove. ☐ ☐ _____

12. Remove the other glove and dispose of it in a facility-approved waste container. ☐ ☐ _____

13. Gather the soiled linens and place them in the linen hamper or linen bag. Dispose of disposable items in a facility-approved waste container. Clean equipment and return it to the storage area. ☐ ☐ _____

14. Take the specimen container to the designated location. ☐ ☐ _____

Finishing Up

15. Complete the "Finishing Up" steps. ☐ ☐ _____

PROCEDURE 23-2
Administering a Soapsuds Enema

Getting Ready	S	U	COMMENTS
1. Complete the "Getting Ready" steps.	☐	☐	_____

Procedure

	S	U	COMMENTS
2. Make sure that the bed is positioned at a comfortable working height (to promote good body mechanics) and that the wheels are locked.	☐	☐	_____
3. Prepare the enema solution in the bathroom or utility room. Clamp the tubing and then fill the enema bag with warm water (105°F [40.5°C] on the bath thermometer) in the specified amount (usually from 500 to 1500 mL). Add the castile soap packet and mix by gently rotating the enema bag. Do not shake the solution vigorously.	☐	☐	_____
4. Release the clamp on the tubing and allow a little water to run through tubing into the sink or bedpan. This will remove all of the air from the tubing. Reclamp the tubing.	☐	☐	_____
5. Hang the enema bag on the IV pole and bring it to the person's bedside. Adjust the height of the IV pole so that the enema bag is hanging no more than 18 inches above the person's anus.	☐	☐	_____
6. If the side rails are in use, lower the side rail on the working side of the bed. The side rail on the opposite side of the bed should remain up. Lower the head of the bed so that the bed is flat (as tolerated).	☐	☐	_____
7. Spread the bath blanket over the top linens (and the person). If the person is able, have her hold the bath blanket. If not, tuck the corners under her shoulders. Fanfold the top linens to the foot of the bed.	☐	☐	_____
8. Ask the person to lie on her left side, facing away from you, in Sims' position. Help her into this position, if necessary.	☐	☐	_____
9. Put on the gloves.	☐	☐	_____
10. Adjust the bath blanket and the person's hospital gown or pajama bottoms as necessary to expose the person's buttocks. Position the bed protector under the person's buttocks to keep the bed linens dry.	☐	☐	_____
11. Open the lubricant package and squeeze a small amount of lubricant onto a paper towel. Lubricate the tip of the enema tubing to ease insertion.	☐	☐	_____

12. Suggest that the person take a deep breath and slowly exhale as the enema tubing is inserted. With one hand, raise the person's upper buttock to expose the anus. Using your other hand, gently and carefully insert the lubricated tip of the tubing into the person's rectum (not more than 3 to 4 inches for adults). Never force the tubing into the rectum. If you are unable to insert the tubing, stop and call the nurse.

13. Unclamp the tubing and allow the solution to begin running. Hold the enema tubing firmly with one hand so that it does not slip out of the rectum. If the person complains of pain or cramping, slow down the rate of flow by tightening the clamp a bit. If the pain or cramping does not stop after slowing the rate of flow, stop the procedure and call the nurse.

14. When the fluid level reaches the bottom of the bag, clamp the tubing to avoid injecting air into the person's rectum.

15. Remove the tubing from the person's rectum and place it inside the enema bag. Gently place several thicknesses of toilet paper against the person's anus to absorb any fluid.

16. Ask the person to retain the enema solution for the specific amount of time.

17. Assist the person with expelling the enema as necessary, using the bedpan, bedside commode, or toilet. If the person is using a regular toilet, ask her not to flush the toilet after expelling the enema.

18. If the person used a regular toilet or bedside commode, assist her with handwashing and then help her to return to bed. Provide perineal care as necessary. If the person used a bedpan, cover and remove the bedpan and assist her with handwashing and perineal care as necessary.

19. Raise the head of the bed as the person requests. Make sure that the bed is lowered to its lowest position and that the wheels are locked. (If the side rails are in use, raise the side rails before leaving the bedside.)

20. Take the covered bedpan or commode bucket (if the person used a bedside commode) to the bathroom.

21. Note the color, amount, and quality of feces before emptying the contents of the bedpan or commode bucket into the toilet. (If anything unusual is observed, do not empty the bedpan or commode bucket until a nurse has had a chance to look at its contents.)

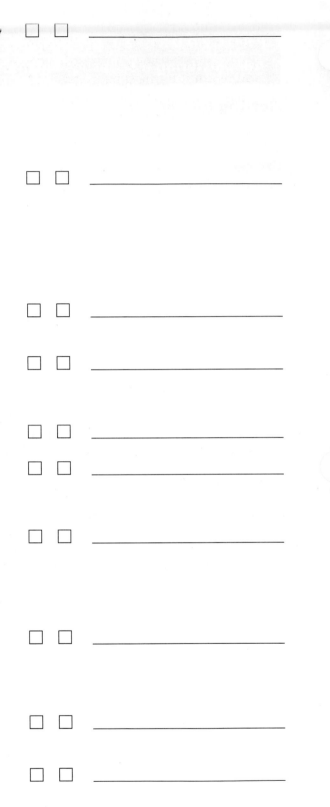

22. Gather the soiled linens and place them in the linen hamper. Dispose of disposable items in a facility-approved waste container. Clean equipment and return it to the storage area.

☐ ☐ _____

23. Remove your gloves and dispose of them in a facility-approved waste container.

☐ ☐ _____

Finishing Up

24. Complete the "Finishing Up" steps.

☐ ☐ _____

PROCEDURE 23-3
Providing Routine Ostomy Care

	S	U	COMMENTS

Getting Ready

1. Complete the "Getting Ready" steps. ☐ ☐ _____

Procedure

2. Cover the over-bed table with paper towels. Place the ostomy supplies and clean linens on the over-bed table. ☐ ☐ _____

3. Make sure that the bed is positioned at a comfortable working height (to promote good body mechanics) and that the wheels are locked. ☐ ☐ _____

4. If the side rails are in use, lower the side rail on the working side of the bed. The side rail on the opposite side of the bed should remain up. If necessary, lower the head of the bed so that the bed is flat (as tolerated). ☐ ☐ _____

5. Fanfold the top linens to below the person's waist. ☐ ☐ _____

6. Position the bed protector on the bed alongside the person to keep the bed linens dry. Adjust the person's clothing as necessary to expose the person's stoma. ☐ ☐ _____

7. Put on the gloves. ☐ ☐ _____

8. Disconnect the ostomy appliance from the ostomy belt if one is used. Remove the belt. If the ostomy belt is soiled, dispose of it in a facility-approved waste container (if it is disposable), or place it in the linen hamper or linen bag (if it is not disposable). ☐ ☐ _____

9. Remove the ostomy appliance by holding the skin taut and gently pulling the appliance away, starting at the top. If the adhesive is making removal difficult, use warm water or the adhesive solvent to soften the adhesive. Place the ostomy appliance in the bedpan. ☐ ☐ _____

10. Gently wipe the stoma with toilet paper to remove any feces or drainage. Place the toilet paper in the bedpan. Cover the stoma with the gauze pad to absorb any drainage that may occur until the new appliance is in place. ☐ ☐ _____

11. Cover the bedpan with the bedpan cover or paper towels. Take the bedpan to the bathroom. (If the side rails are in use, raise them before leaving the bedside.) ☐ ☐ _____

12. Note the color, amount, and quality of the feces before emptying the contents of the ostomy appliance and the bedpan into the toilet. (If anything unusual is observed, do not empty the ostomy appliance until a nurse has had a chance to look at its contents.) ☐ ☐ _____

13. Dispose of the ostomy appliance in a facility-approved waste container. ☐ ☐ _____

14. Remove your gloves and dispose of them in a facility-approved waste container. Wash your hands. ☐ ☐ _____

15. Fill the wash basin with warm water (110°F [43.3°C] to 115°F [46.1°C] on the bath thermometer). Return to the bedside. Place the basin on the over-bed table. If the side rails are in use, lower the side rail on the working side of the bed. ☐ ☐ _____

16. Put on a clean pair of gloves. ☐ ☐ _____

17. Form a mitt around your hand with one of the washcloths. Wet the mitt with warm, clean water and apply soap (or other cleansing agent, per facility policy). Remove the gauze pad from the stoma and dispose of it in a facility-approved waste container. Clean the skin around the stoma. Rinse and dry the skin around the stoma thoroughly. ☐ ☐ _____

18. Apply the skin barrier if needed, according to the manufacturer's directions. ☐ ☐ _____

19. Place the deodorant in the ostomy appliance if deodorant is used. ☐ ☐ _____

20. Put the clean ostomy belt on the person if an ostomy belt is used. ☐ ☐ _____

21. Make sure that the opening on the ostomy appliance is the correct size. Remove the adhesive backing on the ostomy appliance. ☐ ☐ _____

22. Center the appliance over the stoma, making sure that the drain or the end of the bag is pointed down. Gently press around the edges to seal the ostomy appliance to the skin. ☐ ☐ _____

23. Connect the ostomy appliance to the ostomy belt, if one is used. ☐ ☐ _____

24. Remove the bed protector. ☐ ☐ _____

25. Remove your gloves and dispose of them in a facility-approved waste container. ☐ ☐ _____

26. Adjust the person's clothing as necessary to cover the ostomy appliance. If the bedding is wet or soiled, change the bed linens. Help the person back into a comfortable position, straighten the bottom linens, and draw the top linens over the person. Raise the head of the bed, as the person requests. ☐ ☐ _____

27. If the side rails are in use, return the side rail to the raised position. Make sure that the bed is lowered to its lowest position and that the wheels are locked. ☐ ☐ _____

20. Gather the soiled linens and place them in the linen hamper or linen bag. Dispose of disposable items in a facility-approved waste container. Clean equipment and return it to the storage area.

☐ ☐ _____

Finishing Up

29. Complete the "Finishing Up" steps.

☐ ☐ _____

CHAPTER 24 PROCEDURE CHECKLISTS

PROCEDURE 24-1
Giving a Back Massage

	S	U	COMMENTS

Getting Ready

1. Complete the "Getting Ready" steps. ☐ ☐ _____

Procedure

2. Fill the wash basin with warm water. Place the bottle of lotion in the basin of warm water to warm it. ☐ ☐ _____

3. Make sure that the bed is positioned at a comfortable working height (to promote good body mechanics) and that the wheels are locked. ☐ ☐ _____

4. Lower the head of the bed so that the bed is flat (as tolerated). If the side rails are in use, lower the side rail on the working side of the bed. The side rail on the opposite side of the bed should remain up. ☐ ☐ _____

5. Help the person into the prone position, or turn the person onto his side so that he is facing away from you. ☐ ☐ _____

6. Reposition the pillow under the person's head and adjust the bath blanket to keep the person covered, exposing only the back and buttocks. ☐ ☐ _____

7. Put on the gloves if contact with broken skin is likely. ☐ ☐ _____

8. Pour some lotion into your cupped palm and rub your hands together to distribute the lotion onto both palms. ☐ ☐ _____

9. Apply the lotion to the person's back with the palms of your hands. Massage the lotion into the person's skin, using long, gliding strokes (*effleurage*), moving up the center of the back from the buttocks to the shoulders, and then back down along the outside of the back. Do not directly rub any reddened areas. Repeat four times. ☐ ☐ _____

10. For the next set of strokes, move up the center of the back from the buttocks to the shoulders and then back down along the outside of the back. On the downstroke, massage the person's shoulders and back using a small circular motion. Repeat four times. ☐ ☐ _____

11. For the next set of strokes, move up the center of the back from the buttocks to the shoulders, and then back down along the outside of the back. On the downstroke, massage the person's shoulders, back, and buttocks using a small circular motion, paying special attention to the area at the base of the spine. Repeat four times. ☐ ☐ _____

12. Finish with long, gliding strokes (*effleurage*), moving up the center of the back from the buttocks to the shoulders and then back down along the outside of the back. Repeat four times. ☐ ☐ _____

13. Remove your gloves and dispose of them in a facility-approved waste container. ☐ ☐ _____

14. If the back massage is being given as part of a bath, assist the person onto his back and continue with the bath. If the back massage is being given before bed or at any other time, help the person back into his pajamas, nightgown, or hospital gown. ☐ ☐ _____

15. If the side rails are in use, return the side rails to the raised position. Make sure that the bed is lowered to its lowest position and that the wheels are locked. ☐ ☐ _____

16. Gather the soiled linens and place them in the linen hamper or linen bag. Dispose of disposable items in a facility-approved waste container. Clean equipment and return it to the storage area. ☐ ☐ _____

Finishing Up

17. Complete the "Finishing Up" steps. ☐ ☐ _____

PROCEDURE 24-2
Giving a Moist Cold Application

	S	U	COMMENTS

Getting Ready

1. Complete the "Getting Ready" steps. ☐ ☐ _____

Procedure

2. Put the ice in the bath basin and fill the basin with cold water at the sink. ☐ ☐ _____

3. Make sure that the bed is positioned at a comfortable working height (to promote good body mechanics) and that the wheels are locked. ☐ ☐ _____

4. Help the person to a comfortable position and expose only the area to be treated. ☐ ☐ _____

5. Position the bed protector as necessary to keep the bed linens dry. ☐ ☐ _____

6. Moisten the compress with the ice water as ordered. Wring out the compress and apply it to the treatment site. ☐ ☐ _____

7. Leave the compress in place for the designated amount of time, usually 15 to 20 minutes. The compress may be secured in place with ties or rolled gauze, or the patient or resident may assist by holding the compress in place.

    a. Keep the compress moistened with ice water. ☐ ☐ _____

    b. Check the skin beneath the compress every 10 minutes. If the skin appears pale or blue or if the person complains of numbness or a burning sensation, discontinue treatment immediately and notify the nurse. ☐ ☐ _____

    c. If you must leave the room, lower the bed to its lowest position, place the call light control within easy reach and ask the person to signal if she experiences numbness or burning. ☐ ☐ _____

8. When the treatment is complete, remove the compress and carefully dry the skin. ☐ ☐ _____

9. Remove the bed protector. Straighten the bed linens and make sure the person is comfortable and in good body alignment. Draw the top linens over the person. ☐ ☐ _____

10. Make sure that the bed is lowered to its lowest position and that the wheels are locked. ☐ ☐ _____

11. Gather the soiled linens and place them in the linen hamper. Dispose of disposable items in a facility-approved waste container. Clean equipment and return it to the storage area. ☐ ☐ _____

Finishing Up

12. Complete the "Finishing Up" steps. ☐ ☐ _____

PROCEDURE 24-3
Giving a Dry Cold Application

	S	U	COMMENTS

Getting Ready

1. Complete the "Getting Ready" steps. ☐ ☐ _____

Procedure

2. Fill the ice bag with water, close it, and turn it upside down to check for leaks. Empty the bag. ☐ ☐ _____

3. Fill the bag one-half to two-thirds full with crushed ice. Do not overfill the ice bag. Squeeze the bag to force out excess air, and close the bag. ☐ ☐ _____

4. Dry the outside of the bag with the paper towels and wrap it in the towel. ☐ ☐ _____

5. Make sure that the bed is positioned at a comfortable working height (to promote good body mechanics) and that the wheels are locked. ☐ ☐ _____

6. Help the person to a comfortable position and expose only the area to be treated. ☐ ☐ _____

7. Apply the ice bag to the treatment site. Make sure that the towel is in place between the ice bag and the person's skin. ☐ ☐ _____

8. Leave the ice bag in place for the designated amount of time, usually 15 to 20 minutes. The ice bag may be secured in place with ties or rolled gauze, or the patient or resident may assist by holding the ice bag in place.

  a. Check the skin beneath the ice bag every 10 minutes. If the skin appears pale or blue or if the person complains of numbness or a burning sensation, discontinue treatment immediately and notify the nurse. ☐ ☐ _____

  b. Refill the bag with ice as necessary. ☐ ☐ _____

  c. If you must leave the room, lower the bed to its lowest position, place the call light control within easy reach and ask the person to signal if he experiences numbness or burning. ☐ ☐ _____

9. When the treatment is complete, remove the ice bag. ☐ ☐ _____

10. Straighten the bed linens and make sure the person is comfortable and in good body alignment. Draw the top linens over the person. ☐ ☐ _____

11. Make sure that the bed is lowered to its lowest position and that the wheels are locked. ☐ ☐ _____

12. Gather the soiled linens and place them in the linen hamper. Dispose of disposable items in a facility-approved waste container. Clean equipment and return it to the storage area. ☐ ☐ _____

Finishing Up

13. Complete the "Finishing Up" steps. ☐ ☐ _____

PROCEDURE 24-4
Giving a Dry Heat Application With an Aquamatic Pad

	S	U	COMMENTS

Getting Ready

1. Complete the "Getting Ready" steps. ☐ ☐ _____

Procedure

2. Check the pad for leaks. Make sure that the cord is not frayed and the plug is in good condition. Check the heating unit to be sure that it is filled with water. If you need to fill it, use distilled water. Tap water contains minerals that can corrode the unit. ☐ ☐ _____

3. Place the heating unit on a level, firm surface so that the tubing and pad are level with the heating unit at all times. Make sure that the tubing is free of kinks. Plug the cord into an outlet. ☐ ☐ _____

4. Allow the water to warm to the desired temperature, as specified by the nurse or the care plan. If the temperature is not preset, set the temperature with the key and then remove the key. ☐ ☐ _____

5. Place the pad in its cover. ☐ ☐ _____

6. Make sure that the bed is positioned at a comfortable working height (to promote good body mechanics) and that the wheels are locked. ☐ ☐ _____

7. Help the person to a comfortable position and expose only the area to be treated. ☐ ☐ _____

8. Apply the pad to the treatment site. ☐ ☐ _____

9. Leave the pad in place for the designated amount of time, usually 15 to 20 minutes. The pad may be secured in place with ties or tape, or the patient or resident may assist by holding the pad in place. (Do not use pins to secure the pad. Pins can puncture the pad, causing it to leak.)

   a. Check the skin beneath the pad every 5 minutes. If the skin appears red, swollen, or blistered or if the person complains of pain, numbness, or discomfort, discontinue treatment immediately and notify the nurse. ☐ ☐ _____

   b. Refill the heating unit if the water level drops below the fill line. ☐ ☐ _____

   c. If you must leave the room, lower the bed to its lowest position, place the call light control within easy reach and ask the person to signal if she experiences numbness or burning. ☐ ☐ _____

10. When the treatment is complete, remove the pad. ☐ ☐ _____

11. Straighten the bed linens and make sure the person is comfortable and in good body alignment. Draw the top linens over the person. ☐ ☐ _____

12. Make sure that the bed is lowered to its lowest position and that the wheels are locked. ☐ ☐ _____

13. Gather the soiled linens and place them in the linen hamper. Dispose of disposable items in a facility-approved waste container. Clean equipment and return it to the storage area. ☐ ☐ _____

Finishing Up

14. Complete the "Finishing Up" steps. ☐ ☐ _____

CHAPTER 25 PROCEDURE CHECKLISTS

PROCEDURE 25-1
Providing Postmortem Care

Getting Ready	S	U	COMMENTS
1. Complete the "Getting Ready" steps.	☐	☐	_____

Procedure

	S	U	COMMENTS
2. Cover the over-bed table with paper towels. Place your supplies on the over-bed table.	☐	☐	_____
3. Make sure that the bed is positioned at a comfortable working height (to promote good body mechanics) and that the wheels are locked. Lower the head of the bed so that the bed is flat. Fanfold the top linens to the foot of the bed.	☐	☐	_____
4. Put on the gloves.	☐	☐	_____
5. If instructed to by the nurse, remove or turn off any medical equipment.	☐	☐	_____
6. Place the body in the supine position. Position the pillow under the person's head and shoulders. Undress the body and cover it with the bath blanket.	☐	☐	_____
7. Close the eyes. Put a moistened cotton ball on each eyelid if the eyes do not stay closed. If the person has an artificial eye, this should be in place, unless you are instructed otherwise.	☐	☐	_____
8. Replace the person's dentures, unless you are instructed otherwise. Close the mouth and, if necessary, gently support the jaw with the chin strap, a light bandage, or a rolled hand towel.	☐	☐	_____
9. Remove any jewelry and place it in a plastic bag or envelope for the family. List each piece of jewelry as you remove it. Do not remove engagement or wedding rings, unless it is your facility's policy to do so.	☐	☐	_____
10. Fill the wash basin with warm water. Place the basin on the over-bed table. Wash the body and comb the hair.	☐	☐	_____
11. If the family is to view the body, dress the body in a clean gown. If the bedding is wet or soiled, change the bed linens. Draw the top linens over the person, forming a cuff at the shoulders. (Do not cover the person's face.) Straighten the room, lower the lights, and provide for the family's privacy.	☐	☐	_____
12. After the family leaves, collect all of the person's belongings, noting each item on your list.	☐	☐	_____

13. Fill out three identification tags:

    a. Attach one to the right great toe or the right ankle. ☐ ☐ _____

    b. Attach one to the person's belongings. ☐ ☐ _____

    c. Save the last to be attached to the outside of the shroud (if used). ☐ ☐ _____

14. If a shroud is to be used, apply it now and attach the third identification tag to the outside of the shroud. ☐ ☐ _____

15. Gather the soiled linens and place them in the linen hamper. Dispose of disposable items in a facility-approved waste container. Clean equipment and return it to the storage area. ☐ ☐ _____

16. Remove your gloves and dispose of them in a facility-approved waste container. ☐ ☐ _____

17. Transfer the body from the bed to a stretcher for transport to the morgue, if appropriate. If the family has made funeral arrangements, leave the body in the room with the door or curtain closed. ☐ ☐ _____

18. Report the time the body was transported and the location of the person's belongings to the nurse. ☐ ☐ _____

Finishing Up

19. Complete the "Finishing Up" steps. ☐ ☐ _____

CHAPTER 30 PROCEDURE CHECKLISTS

PROCEDURE 30-1
Applying Anti-Embolism (TED) Stockings

	S	U	COMMENTS

Getting Ready

1. Complete the "Getting Ready" steps. ☐ ☐ _____

Procedure

2. Make sure that the bed is positioned at a comfortable working height (to promote good body mechanics) and that the wheels are locked. If the side rails are in use, lower the side rail on the working side of the bed. The side rail on the opposite side of the bed should remain up. ☐ ☐ _____

3. Help the person into the supine position. ☐ ☐ _____

4. Fanfold the top linens to the foot of the bed. Adjust the person's hospital gown or pajama bottoms as necessary to expose one leg at a time. ☐ ☐ _____

5. Turn the stocking inside out down to the heel. ☐ ☐ _____

6. Slip the foot of the stocking over the person's toes, foot, and heel. The stocking has an opening in the toe area, which allows the health care team to assess the person's toes to make sure they are receiving enough blood. Depending on the manufacturer, this opening may be on the top or on the bottom of the stocking. ☐ ☐ _____

7. Grasp the top of the stocking and pull it up the person's leg. The stocking will turn itself right-side out as you pull it up the person's leg. ☐ ☐ _____

8. Check to make sure that the stocking is not twisted and that it fits snugly against the person's leg, with no wrinkles. Also make sure that the stocking fits smoothly over the heel and that the opening in the toe area is correctly located in the toe region. ☐ ☐ _____

9. Cover that leg, expose the other leg, and repeat steps 5 through 8. ☐ ☐ _____

10. Help the person back into a comfortable position, straighten the bottom linens, and draw the top linens over the person. Raise the head of the bed as the person requests. Make sure that the bed is lowered to its lowest position and that the wheels are locked. ☐ ☐ _____

Finishing Up

11. Complete the "Finishing Up" steps. ☐ ☐ _____

NOTES

NOTES

NOTES

NOTES

NOTES

NOTES

NOTES

NOTES

NOTES

NOTES

NOTES